Waking up to the morning-after pill

Waking up to the morning-after pill

How parents are being undermined by the promotion of emergency hormonal birth control to under-16s

Norman Wells and Helena Hayward

FAMILY EDUCATION TRUST

FAMILY EDUCATION TRUST
First published 2007

© Family Education Trust, 2007
ISBN (10) 0-906229-19-7
ISBN (13) 978-0-906229-19-4

Family Education Trust
Jubilee House
19-21 High Street
Whitton
Twickenham
TW2 7LB
email: fyc@ukfamily.org.uk
website: www.famyouth.org.uk

Family Education Trust is a company limited by guarantee
(No 3503533) and a registered charity (No 1070500).

Printed in Great Britain by Redlin Print Limited, Chelmsford, Essex

Contents

A note on terms used

The subject of this book is designated in a variety of ways. In common parlance it is widely referred to as the 'morning-after pill' and its manufacturers describe it as an 'emergency contraceptive', while journal articles frequently add the word 'hormonal' in order to distinguish it from the intra-uterine device (IUD) which is intended to serve the identical purpose of preventing the implantation of a fertilised egg in the womb lining.

The 'emergency hormonal pill' is not therefore a conventional contraceptive in that it is intended to act after rather than before conception. For this reason, it can more accurately be described as 'emergency hormonal birth control' (EHBC). This is therefore the term we have chosen to use, though inevitably in the course of quoting from other sources, other designations will appear, of which 'emergency contraception' and 'the morning-after pill' are the most common.

Glossary of acronyms

BMA	British Medical Association
BMJ	British Medical Journal
BPAS	British Pregnancy Advisory Service
CSM	Committee on Safety of Medicines
DfEE	Department for Education and Employment
EC	Emergency contraception
EHBC	Emergency hormonal birth control
EHC	Emergency hormonal contraception
FFPRHC	Faculty of Family Planning and Reproductive Health Care
FDA	Food and Drugs Administration
fpa	Family Planning Association
GMC	General Medical Council
GUM	Genitourinary medicine
LCPC	London Child Protection Committee
LES	Locally Enhanced Service
MHRA	Medicines and Healthcare products Regulatory Agency
MSI	Marie Stopes International
PNA	Pharmaceutical Needs Assessment
PCT	Primary Care Trust
PGD	Patient Group Direction.
POEC	Progesterone-only emergency contraception
RPSGB	Royal Pharmaceutical Society of Great Britain
SPC	Summary of Product Characteristics
SPUC	Society for the Protection of Unborn Children
SRE	Sex and relationships education
STI	Sexually transmitted infection
TIC-TAC	Teenage Information Centre, Teenage Advice Centre

Executive Summary

- Emergency hormonal birth control (EHBC) has been surrounded by controversy since it was first approved for use in the UK during the 1980s. Since then, in a series of unparalleled moves, it has been made available off-prescription for general rather than exceptional use, sold to women over the age of 16 in pharmacies, and supplied to girls under the legal age of consent to sexual intercourse in a variety of settings.

- The government is committed to making EHBC more widely available to teenage girls as a major strand of its teenage pregnancy strategy.

- Both the manufacturers and the government insist that EHBC does not produce an abortion. However, very real ethical issues remain, since the only way it can be claimed that EHBC is not abortifacient is by redefining the meaning of conception.

- In order to make EHBC available to girls under the age of 16, it has been necessary to set professional concerns aside. The original assessment report made no specific assessment of the safety of EHBC for girls aged 15 and under. The Summary of Product Characteristics for the prescription-only product states that the drug 'is not recommended in children' and that 'very limited data are available' to support its use by under-16s.

- The availability of EHBC on school premises runs counter to the government's good practice guide with regard to the supply of medical treatment in schools.

- Since EHBC became available off-prescription, the proportion of women obtaining it from pharmacies has risen rapidly. The provision of EHBC under Patient Group Directions (PGDs) is one of the government's public health priorities as a means of reducing the under-18 conception rate and improving sexual health.

- PGDs permitting the supply of EHBC to girls under the age of consent are in place in 128 Primary Care Trusts (PCTs) in England (84 per cent of the total).

- Many PCTs are using the National Health Service (Pharmaceutical Services) Regulations 2005 as a mechanism to force new pharmacies to supply EHBC to girls under the age of 16. Of the 128 PCTs with PGDs, 90 (70 per cent) indicated that, under some circumstances, they would insist on the provision of EHBC to underage girls as a condition of granting a pharmacy licence.

- The majority of PCTs cite high teenage pregnancy rates and the government's teenage pregnancy strategy as the rationale for issuing PGDs permitting the supply of EHBC to girls under the age of 16, but not a single PCT made any attempt to cite research evidence linking easy access to EHBC with a reduction in teenage pregnancy rates.

- There is evidence that the perceived reduction in risk afforded by making contraception and EHBC readily available to young people may be encouraging a more casual attitude to sex and removing one of the major restraints to underage sexual activity. When introducing measures aimed at reducing teenage conception rates, it is important to consider the impact of those measures on the behaviour of young people themselves.

- There are particular health risks associated with the supply of EHBC to girls under the age of 16 in pharmacies and in other settings where their full medical history is not known. The easier it is to obtain EHBC in confidence, the more scope there is for the exploitation and abuse of young people.

- Making EHBC available to girls under the age of consent to sexual intercourse conveys the message that there is nothing wrong with sex at any age, that actions need not have lasting consequences, and that there is a drug to deal with every eventuality.

- Many health professionals appeal to criteria laid down by Lord Fraser in his ruling in the Gillick case as the legal basis for the confidential provision of contraception to children under the age of consent. Few are aware that Lord Fraser went on to stress that these criteria 'ought not to be regarded as a licence for doctors to disregard the wishes of parents on this matter whenever they find it convenient to do so'.

- There is perhaps no other area on which the government presents breaking the law as an option and even helps to facilitate lawbreaking as it does in relation to the confidential provision of contraception to young people under the age of consent to sexual intercourse.

- Some medical bodies and contraceptive advocacy groups are so committed to the principle of confidentiality that they are prepared to bypass established child protection procedures. The British Medical Association, General Medical Council, Brook, *fpa*, and the Office of the Commissioner for Children and Young People are among bodies strongly opposed to the mandatory reporting of sexually active under-13s.

- Despite the absence of any evidence that supplying contraception and EHBC to girls under the age of 16 on school premises reduces teenage pregnancy or abortion rates, Department of Health guidance encourages school nurses to provide and promote confidential drop-ins, and Ofsted regards the provision of EHBC on school premises as 'a valuable service'.

- Advocates of confidential contraceptive services claim they are beneficial because without the guarantee of confidentiality young people would not seek advice. However, in the United States teenage conception and abortion rates have declined more rapidly in areas where mandatory parental notification laws have been in place.

- While the government trumpets the importance of parents in reducing teenage conception rates, its confidentiality policy undermines and marginalises them. The more the state undermines the authority of parents, the less responsibility parents will be inclined to take for their children.

- Rather than persisting with an approach that is failing in the hope that it may 'come good' in the process of time, PCTs should undertake an honest appraisal of their policies regarding the supply of EHBC to under-16s in line with the evidence.

- In the absence of any evidence that EHBC leads to a reduction in under-16 conceptions, it is untenable for PCTs to insist on supply to underage girls as a condition of granting a pharmacy licence.

- Pharmacies, supermarket chains and schools which are currently supplying EHBC to girls below the age of 16 under a PGD should review their policies and consider the possibility that they may be adding to the problems associated with underage sexual activity rather than contributing to the solution.
- Rather than continuing to formulate policy on the assumption that teenagers will engage in sexual activity irrespective of anything parents and teachers say to them, we need to recognise that the majority of young people under the age of 16 are not sexually active, and to support and affirm them in their exercise of self-control. Until we overcome our current phobia about abstinence and our obsession with sexual expression, we are unlikely to make any real progress.

1. Setting the scene

The 'morning-after pill', more accurately described as emergency hormonal birth control (EHBC), has been surrounded by controversy since it was first approved for use in the UK during the 1980s. At that time, the then Department of Health and Social Security offered assurances that it would be used only in exceptional circumstances, and that it would remain as a prescription-only drug under the control of doctors.

However, in a series of unparalleled moves, EHBC became available for general, rather than exceptional, use. It has become available off-prescription, sold to women over the age of 16 in pharmacies, and made available to girls under the legal age of consent to sexual intercourse in a variety of settings. Advance supply of EHBC has been approved by the professional and regulatory body for pharmacists in Great Britain, many Primary Care Trusts (PCTs) are insisting on its provision to girls below the age of 16 as a condition of granting a pharmacy licence, the rate of VAT charged on purchases has been reduced from 17.5 per cent to five per cent, and there are even calls for it to be made available to men seeking to obtain it on behalf of their sexual partners.[1]

The government is committed to making EHBC more widely available to teenage girls as part of its efforts to halve the number of conceptions among under-18s by 2010. In 2001, the then Health Minister Jacqui Smith stated: 'Improving teenagers' access to contraceptive advice, including emergency contraception, is a key strand of the government's teenage pregnancy strategy.'[2] This strategy includes making EHBC readily available to those under the legal age of consent to sexual intercourse.

What is EHBC and how does it work?

Prior to the year 2000, the only form of EHBC available in the UK was a combined pill, so called because it contained oestrogen and progestogen, the two hormones commonly found in the contraceptive pill. However, in the Autumn of 1999, a new progestogen-only drug, levonorgestrel

---

[1] Levenson E, 'Allow men to take more responsibility for sex', *Independent*, 30 December 2006.
[2] HC Deb (2000-01) 363, written answers col.663.

(Levonelle-2), was licensed for use in the UK and became available on prescription from February 2000. It was claimed that the lack of an oestrogen component in Levonelle-2 would make oral emergency contraception accessible to women for whom the earlier pill was not advised.[3] Health experts throughout the world heralded the progestogen-only pill as safer, more effective and carrying with it fewer side-effects. The prescription-only medicine, Levonelle-2 (two tablets containing 750 micrograms of levonorgestrel), has since been discontinued and replaced by Levonelle 1500 (a single tablet containing 1500 micrograms of levonorgestrel). The pharmacy-only drug is an identical product to Levonelle 1500 and known as Levonelle One Step.[4]

The stated purpose of EHBC is to prevent an unwanted pregnancy after intercourse has taken place. The manufacturer of the licensed drug describes it as: 'an emergency contraceptive that can be used after un-protected sex or where a contraceptive method has failed. This type of contraception is often called "the morning-after pill"'.[5]

It is not known precisely how EHBC works. The manufacturers state that Levonelle-2 is thought to work by:

- stopping your ovaries from releasing an egg;

- preventing sperm from fertilising any egg you may have already released; or

- stopping a fertilised egg from attaching itself to your womb lining.[6]

Ethical considerations

Both the manufacturers and the government are insistent that EHBC does not produce an abortion and that 'it does not work if you are already pregnant'.[7] However, these oft-repeated assurances mask a very real ethical issue. The only way in which it can be claimed that EHBC is incapable of acting as an abortifacient is by redefining the meaning of conception.

---

[3] UK Drug Information Pharmacists Group, New Medicines on the Market: Levonorgestrel, 1999.

[4] In the United States, EHBC consists of two tablets containing 750 micrograms of levonorgestrel, akin to Levonelle-2 which has now been discontinued in the UK. It is licensed as a single product, with pharmacy supply limited to women aged 18 and over, while a prescription is required for supply to young women aged 17 and under. Both classifications are marketed as Plan B.

[5] Schering, Patient Information Leaflets for both Levonelle 1500 and Levonelle One Step.

[6] ibid

[7] ibid

According to established biological definition, the word 'conception' refers to the point at which the sperm meets the egg and fertilises it. *Contra*ception works to prevent this, whether by physical or chemical means. Where EHBC operates to stop or delay the ovaries from releasing an egg, or to prevent sperm from fertilising an egg, it is acting as a contraceptive. However, where the pill functions to stop a fertilised egg from attaching itself to the womb lining, it is not serving as a contraceptive because conception has already taken place.

In 1983, the Attorney-General ruled that EHBC did not constitute a criminal offence under the Offences Against the Person Act 1861, which forbids any action which has the intent of procuring a miscarriage.[8] He considered that prior to the implantation of the embryo in the lining of the womb, five or six days after conception, 'carriage' cannot have occurred, and that the use of a pill which operated prior to implantation could not be deemed to procure a 'miscarriage' under the terms of the 1861 Act.

It is on the basis of this advice that successive governments have taken the view that 'a pregnancy begins at implantation' (rather than at conception) and can refer to this as 'the accepted legal and medical view'.[9] It also cleared the way to licence the emergency pill as a 'contraceptive'.

The debate continues, however. In November 2001, the Advertising Standards Authority ruled that an advertisement placed in several newspapers by the Society for the Protection of Unborn Children (SPUC) was 'misleading' because it went against 'the accepted legal and medical view' when it claimed that EHBC was 'abortion inducing'. SPUC were advised that if they persisted with the advertisement, they could be referred to the Office of Fair Trading and face penalties.[10]

In a subsequent Judicial Review hearing, SPUC argued that the prescription and supply of EHBC constituted a breach of the Offences Against the Person Act 1861, since the meaning of the word 'miscarriage' included the expulsion of an unimplanted embryo when the Act was framed. However, in his judgment, Justice Munby determined that his decision must rest not on the meaning of the word 'miscarriage' in 1861, but on its meaning today, which he considered had to do with

---

[8] *Official Report*, 10 May 1983; Vol. 42, c. 237, cited in HC Deb (1999-2000) 357, written answers col.470.
[9] HC Deb (1999-2000) 357, written answers col.354.
[10] Advertising Standards Authority, www.asa.org.uk Case no: A01-06470/PJ.
[11] Smeaton v Secretary of State for Health [2002] EWHC 610 (Admin) (18 April 2002)

'the termination of an established pregnancy, and there is no established pregnancy prior to implantation'. He thus dismissed the case advanced by SPUC on the basis that there was no evidence that EHBC caused the loss of a fertilised egg after implantation.[11]

Dr John Ling, formerly of the Institute of Biological Sciences at Aberystwyth University, refers to the current legal position in terms of a 'new biology' whereby, contrary to centuries of biological scholarship, conception has been separated from fertilisation. He describes it as an example of lexical engineering preceding social engineering.[12] It remains a simple matter of fact that the embryo is contained and 'carried' within the womb irrespective of whether implantation has taken place.

The feminist author Germaine Greer is in no doubt that EHBC is an abortifacient and considers it deceptive and undermining to the dignity of women to conceal the fact:

> These days, contraception is abortion because...pills cannot be shown to prevent sperm fertilising an ovum... Whether you feel that the creation and wastage of so many embryos is an important issue or not, you must see that the cynical deception of women by selling abortifacients as if they were contraceptives is incompatible with the respect due to women as human beings.[13]

How effective is it?

Measuring the effectiveness of EHBC is extremely complex for the simple reason that, when it is taken, there is no way of ascertaining whether conception has taken place. Women who take EHBC do so as a precautionary measure rather than on the basis of any sure knowledge of a developing pregnancy.

A World Health Organisation study which estimated the number of anticipated pregnancies, taking into account the menstrual and sexual histories of participating women, and then compared them with the actual numbers of pregnancies occurring after treatment, found that the effectiveness of EHBC varied considerably depending on how soon after intercourse it was taken (Table 1).[14]

---

[12] Ling J R. *Responding to the Culture of Death*, London: Day One, 2001.

[13] Greer G. *The Whole Woman*, London: Doubleday, 1999, pp92-93.

[14] Task Force on Postovulatory Methods of Fertility Regulation, 'Randomised controlled trial of levonorgestrel versus the Yuzpe regimen of combined oral contraceptives for emergency contraception', *Lancet* 1998; 352:428-433.

Table 1: Effectiveness of progestogen-only emergency hormonal birth control

Interval between intercourse and treatment	
24 hours or less	95%
25-48 hours	85%
49-72 hours	58%

Source: Lancet 1998; 352:428-433

However, a more recent systematic review published in the journal of *Obstetrics and Gynecology* suggests that the effectiveness of EHBC may have been over-stated. Referring to an analysis of the effectiveness of the emergency pill, the authors suggest that, 'we can be 95 per cent confident that it reduces pregnancy risk by more than 23 per cent', but go on to add that figures suggesting an average rate of effectiveness around 80 per cent 'may overstate actual efficacy, possibly quite substantially'.[15]

Government investment in EHBC

In its attempt to prevent unwanted pregnancies and reduce the teenage pregnancy rate, the government is continuing to invest heavily in contraceptive services in general and in EHBC in particular. In addition to its funding of the teenage pregnancy strategy, it has pledged £40 million over two years (£20 million in both 2006/07 and 2007/08) to enable PCTs to 'improve access to contraceptive services and to the full range of methods'.[16]

During 2006 the cost to the NHS of providing EHBC under prescription amounted to £2.2 million in England (Figure 1). This sum does not include EHBC supplied by community contraception clinics or issued under Patient Group Directions.[17] It does not therefore take account of the growing numbers of young people who are obtaining EHBC free of charge from local pharmacies and contraception clinics.

---

[15] Raymond E G, Trussell, J, Polis C B, 'Population Effect of Increased Access to Emergency Contraceptive Pill', *Obstetrics and Gynecology*, Vol 109, No 1, January 2007.

[16] HC Deb (2005-06) 446, written answers, col 2014.

[17] HC Deb (2006-07) 463, written answers, col 979.

Figure 1: Cost to the NHS of prescriptions for EHBC dispensed in the community: England, 1999-2006

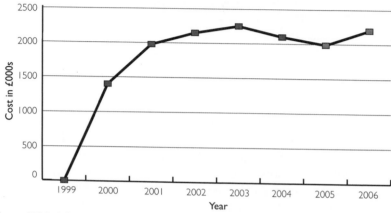

Source: HC Deb (2006–07), 463, written answers, col 979.

In 2006, GPs prescribed 280,600 items of EHBC, while 164,500 women obtained emergency pills from community contraception clinics.[18] The number of girls and women who obtained EHBC over the counter in pharmacies is not known, but figures from an Office for National Statistics omnibus survey suggests that 45 per cent of women accessing EHBC obtain it from pharmacies, compared with 30 per cent from GPs, and 24 per cent from community contraception clinics (Figure 2).[19]

Figure 2: Where EHBC is obtained, Great Britain, 2005-2006:
Women aged 16-49 who had used the emergency pill in the year prior to interview

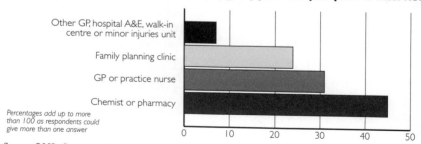

Source: ONS, Contraception and Sexual Health, 2005/06

[18] HC Deb (2006-07) 463, written answers, col 1356.
[19] ONS, *Contraception and Sexual Health, 2005/06*, Omnibus Survey Report No 30.

2. Getting the emergency pill off-prescription

During the Spring of 2000, the manufacturers submitted an application for the reclassification of the prescription-only status of Levonelle-2 to make it available in pharmacies.[1] At the same time, the Council minutes of the Royal Pharmaceutical Society of Great Britain (RPSGB) noted that 'there was now wide acceptance that pharmacists had a role to play in helping reduce the numbers of unwanted pregnancies by supplying EHC' and welcomed the prospect of a pharmacy product for EHBC.[2]

It was originally envisaged that the change in classification would require ratification by Parliament after approval by health ministers, but, in the event, the government introduced two measures without parliamentary debate which had the effect of making Levonelle-2 available without a doctor's prescription.

Firstly, in August 2000, Patient Group Directions (PGDs) were introduced in various parts of the UK to allow nurses, pharmacists and other health workers to administer or supply prescription-only medicines, as specified by local health authorities, without a doctor's prescription.[3] This provision made it possible for family planning clinics and health workers, including school nurses, to supply EHBC to women and girls of all ages, and pilot schemes offering emergency contraception over-the-counter, free of charge, were operated by pharmacies in areas with high unwanted pregnancy rates.[4]

Secondly, in December 2000, the government laid a second Order before Parliament, which permitted progestogen-only EHBC to be sold over-the-counter at pharmacies to women aged 16 and over. By-passing

---

[1] Committee on Safety of Medicines, Summary of the Committee on Safety and Medicines meeting held on Thursday 23 March 2000.

[2] RPSGB Council Minutes, 4 April 2000. Extracts from RPSGB Council Minutes and other internal documents referred to were obtained under the provisions of the Freedom of Information Act 2000.

[3] SI 2000 No 1917 *The Prescription Only Medicines (Human Use) Amendment Order 2000*. The Department of Health describes PGDs as 'documents which make it legal for medicines to be given to groups of patients… without individual prescriptions having to be written for each patient. They can also be used to empower staff other than doctors…to legally give the medicine in question.'

[4] Harrison-Woolrych M, Duncan A, Howe J, Smith C, 'Improving access to emergency contraception', *BMJ* 2001; 322:186-187.

the convention that 40 days should be allowed for parliamentary scrutiny and debate, the government chose to bring the measure into force on 1 January 2001 without public consultation or parliamentary debate.[5] One enthusiastic supporter of the move later hailed it as 'another great leap forward for womankind'.[6]

In the meantime, the RPSGB Council considered an Expert Advisory Group report on 'Advice on best practice in the supply of Emergency Hormonal Contraception as a Pharmacy medicine' and approved five professional standards for the sale of EHBC as a pharmacy medicine. These standards were subsequently incorporated into the Society's 'best practice' guidance which was published in advance of EHBC being made available in pharmacies from the beginning of 2001. The five standards required that:

(a) Pharmacists must deal with the request personally and decide whether to supply the product or refer the patient to an appropriate healthcare professional;

(b) Pharmacists must ensure that all necessary advice and information is provided to enable the patient to assess whether to use the product;

(c) Requests for emergency hormonal contraception should be handled sensitively with due regard being given to the patient's right to privacy;

(d) Only in exceptional circumstances should pharmacists supply the product to a person other than the patient;

(e) Pharmacists should whenever possible take reasonable measures to inform patients of regular methods of contraception, disease prevention and sources of help.[7]

The guidance stated that, having obtained and assessed the relevant information, the pharmacist may feel EHBC was not needed. However, if the woman perceived herself at risk of pregnancy and, despite the pharmacist's professional advice, still wished to take the drug, then in the absence of any obvious contraindication, the pharmacist should consider supplying it to her. The guidance proceeded to suggest that:

---

[5] SI 2000 No 3231 *The Prescription Only Medicines (Human Use) Amendment (No 3) Order 2000.*
[6] HL Deb (2006-07) 691, col 482.
[7] Royal Pharmaceutical Society, 'Practice guidance on the supply of Emergency Hormonal Contraception as a pharmacy medicine', December 2000, para 2.1.

EHC poses very little safety risk to clients, even if taken when not necessary... If a client inadvertently takes EHC when she is already pregnant, she should be reassured that EHC is not an abortifacient, does not appear to pose a risk to pregnancy, nor does it appear to harm the baby. It is important to note that no guarantee can be given about any pregnancy whether EHC is used or not.[8]

In response to the public controversy that surrounded the decision to make EHBC available in pharmacies, an open letter was issued by the President of the RSPGB together with senior officers of the Royal College of General Practitioners, the General Practitioners Committee and the Royal College of Nursing. The letter concluded:

We believe that the wider access through pharmacies to progestogen-only EHC will complement the existing routes of supply and is a responsible and socially beneficial development that should be allowed to establish itself in the name of the greater good.[9]

EHBC and under-16s

It is worthy of note that in the original assessment report generated by the Medicines and Healthcare products Regulatory Agency (MHRA) no specific assessment was made of the safety of Levonelle-2 for girls under the age of 16.[10] This is reflected in the Summary of Product Characteristics (SPC) for the prescription-only product. The SPC states that the drug 'is not recommended in children', adding that 'very limited data are available' to support its use by under-16s.[11]

In its consideration of an application to reclassify EHBC from being a prescription-only drug to make it available from pharmacies, the

---

[8] *ibid.*, paras 4.4, 17. While the RPSGB was sanguine with regard to the effect of EHBC upon a developing baby, the medical assessment report prepared by the Medicines and Healthcare products Regulatory Agency was more cautious: 'Although emergency contraception with levonorgestrel is effective, some pregnancies do occur and the possibility of ectopic pregnancy or birth defects are of particular concern. In general, among women taking oral contraceptives daily, the proportion of pregnancies that are ectopic is greater for progestogen-only pills than for combined oral contraceptives.' Medicines and Healthcare products Regulatory Agency, Medical Assessment of Levonelle-2 750 Microgram Tablet (PL 0527/0016). Information relating to the assessment during the licensing process was obtained from MHRA under the provisions of the Freedom of Information Act 2000.

[9] An open letter from the Royal College of General Practitioners, the General Practitioners Committee of the British Medical Association, the Royal College of Nursing and the Royal Pharmaceutical Society of Great Britain, 'Emergency hormonal contraception as a Pharmacy product', 25 January 2001.

[10] Medicines and Healthcare products Regulatory Agency, Medical Assessment of Levonelle-2 750, *op. cit.*

[11] Bayer Schering, Summary of Product Characteristics for Levonelle 1500.
http://www.emc.medicines.org.uk/emc/assets/c/html/displaydoc.asp?documentid=16887

Committee on Safety of Medicines (CSM) took the view that provision of the emergency pill presented 'special risk management issues' and concluded that, 'because of the likelihood of these possible indirect dangers to health in those under 16 years of age', it should not be supplied to those in that category without medical supervision. The Committee also noted that 16 is the legal age of consent to sexual intercourse.[12]

Notwithstanding these professional concerns, in its practice guidance the Royal Pharmaceutical Society insisted that girls under the age of 16 were entitled to a sympathetic and confidential consultation. In the absence of a PGD permitting pharmacy supply to underage girls, the Society encouraged pharmacists to assist them to obtain EHBC by another route.[13]

The following summer, in its national strategy for sexual health and HIV, the Department of Health claimed that, in some areas, pilot schemes for the provision of 'emergency contraception', pregnancy testing and other aspects of sexual health had proved successful. The Department proposed to issue guidance on expanding NHS provision of 'emergency contraception' in pharmacies.

Under a section on 'Improving practice', the strategy document noted that Manchester, Salford & Trafford, and Lambeth, Southwark & Lewisham Health Action Zones had developed innovative schemes where community pharmacists supplied EHBC using a PGD. The document went on to state that pharmacies were an important additional access route for EHBC, particularly at weekends and bank holidays when other services might not be available. Under these schemes pharmacies had worked with local GPs, family planning clinics, youth clinics and NHS Direct to agree clear standards derived from professional guidelines. The strategy document recommended that 'as a minimum, all walk-in centres should offer emergency contraception and respond to other urgent needs'.[14]

Growing numbers of Primary Care Trusts issued PGDs making EHBC readily available to underage girls without a doctor's prescription. The terms of PGDs varied from region to region but in some areas EHBC became available to girls of any age. For example, in a magazine

---

[12] Committee on Safety of Medicines, *op. cit.*
[13] Royal Pharmaceutical Society, 'Practice guidance', *op. cit.*, paras 10.1, 11.2.
[14] Department of Health, *The national strategy for sexual health and HIV,* July 2001.

distributed to all households in its area, East Surrey Health Authority advised residents that the local hospital offers 'an "all day, every day service" where emergency contraception can be obtained confidentially and free of charge *by girls of any age*' (emphasis added).[15] Girls as young as 12 were able to obtain EHBC at the Magic Roundabout in Kingston-upon-Thames. This self-referral, confidential sexual health advice service targeted at young people aged 12-20 was commended by the government's report on teenage pregnancy as a 'promising approach'.[16]

Schools

Under a PGD, school nurses may also supply EHBC to girls under the age of 16 at the discretion of school governing bodies, in consultation with parents and the school community.[17] However, the availability of EHBC in schools runs counter to the government's good practice guide with regard to the supply of medical treatment in schools. Official guidance states that:

- 'Parents or guardians have prime responsibility for their child's health and should provide schools with information about their child's medical condition.'

- 'Parents' cultural and religious views should always be respected.'

- There should be 'prior written agreement from parents or guardians for any medication, prescribed or non-prescription, to be given to a child'.

- 'School staff should generally not give non-prescribed medication to pupils [e.g. aspirin and paracetamol]. They may not know whether the pupil has taken a previous dose, or whether the medication may react with other medication being taken.'

- 'No pupil under the age of 16 should be given medication without his or her parent's written consent.'[18]

This guidance has been completely overlooked in connection with the supply of EHBC in the school context, with full government support as part of its plan to 'modernise' school nursing services.

---

[15] East Surrey Health Authority, *Care Spectrum*, Spring 2001.
[16] Social Exclusion Unit. *Teenage Pregnancy*, London: HMSO, 1999.
[17] HC Deb (1999-2000) 357, written answers, cols.47-48.
[18] Department for Education & Employment, Department of Health. *Supporting Pupils with Medical Needs: A good practice guide*, London: HMSO 1996.

A report from the Chief Nursing Officer referred positively to a pilot project undertaken by secondary schools across four PCTs with higher than average rates of teenage pregnancy involving the provision of EHBC by school nurses. The same report commended an 'innovative' approach taken by a PCT covering a rural area whereby an arrangement is in place with a local General Practice to allow the school nurse a facility to undertake screening for STIs [sexually transmitted infections] and to offer EHBC under a PGD.[19]

Advance supply

The Family Planning Association (now known as *fpa*) has long been positive about advance supply of EHBC. In response to the question, 'Can I get emergency pills in advance?' the Association confidently answers, 'Yes, if you are going on holiday or are worried about your contraceptive method failing. Ask your doctor or family planning clinic about this.'[20] However, until relatively recently the professional and regulatory body for pharmacists in Britain was more cautious.

In December 2000, the Royal Pharmaceutical Society's guidance to pharmacists stated that:

Supply of emergency hormonal contraception (EHC) via the pharmacy in advance of need is not currently recommended. Clients requesting advance supplies should be advised that some, but not all, doctors and family planning services may prescribe EHC for advance situations. Pharmacists should ensure that they know if and where this is provided locally so that the information can be offered to clients.[21]

An unpublished report prepared for the RPSGB by an Expert Advisory Group which included the Director of Information at the *fpa* had come short of recommending advance supply 'at this stage', but expressed the belief that 'this situation may change with experience and should be reviewed at a later date'.[22]

[19] Children's Workforce Unit, Department for Education and Skills, *Chief Nursing Officer's Programme for School Nursing – Examples of School Nursing Practice*, September 2005
http://www.everychildmatters.gov.uk/_files/EF39C790B51F4C47EC9FB8548010BF18.doc
[20] Family Planning Association. Emergency Contraception,
http://www.fpa.org.uk/information/leaflets/documents_and_pdfs/detail.cfm?contentID=141
[21] Royal Pharmaceutical Society. 'Practice guidance', op. cit., para 12.1, emphasis added.
[22] RPSGB Expert Advisory Group report on Emergency Hormonal Contraception, 'Advice on best practice in the supply of Emergency Hormonal Contraception as a Pharmacy medicine', September 2000.

The question of advance supply was accordingly kept under review and, in April 2003, following internal discussions, the RPSGB Practice Committee proposed a review of the guidance with a view to removing the recommendation against advance supply. It had come to the Society's attention, via the manufacturer of levonorgestrel, that some clients were lying to pharmacists in order to obtain advance supply. Some product users had written to the manufacturer objecting to the need to do this in order to obtain the drug in advance. Under 'points for consideration' it was noted that advance supply would 'help in meeting the government's goal for teenage pregnancy' and that the *fpa* had a policy that women should be able to obtain EHBC in advance of need.[23]

Six months later, the Practice Committee of the RPSGB recommended a change of policy on advance supply 'in the light of recent developments'. The only research evidence advanced in support of the recommendation was a study published in *Obstetrics and Gynecology* which had concluded that 'advance provision of emergency contraception significantly increased use without adversely affecting use of routine contraception'. The authors of the study then proceeded to demonstrate their unbounded zeal for EHBC promotion by recommending that it should be supplied to all mothers when they returned home with their newborn babies:

> It is safe and appropriate to provide emergency contraception to all postpartum women before discharge from hospital.[24]

The following proposition was accordingly laid before the RPSGB Council at its meeting in December 2003:

> Mindful of the fact that FP [family planning] professionals were already involved in advance supply, Practice Division wished to update the existing guidance to take account of recent developments and evidence-based research.

After a brief discussion, the RPSGB Council in closed business resolved:

> that practice guidance on supply of EC be reviewed with particular consideration to removing the recommendation against advance supply.

---

[23] Royal Pharmaceutical Society Practice Committee document on 'Advance supply of Emergency Hormonal Contraception (Levonorgestrel – P medicine)', April 2003.

[24] Jackson RA; Schwarz B; Freedman L; Darney P, 'Advance supply of emergency contraception effect use and usual contraception – a randomised trial', *Obstetrics and Gynecology* 2003; 102 (issue 1); 8-16 July.

At the request of the Department of Health and the MHRA, a meeting was held in June 2004 to discuss issues concerning advance supply and updates to the RPSGB's Practice Guidance. Three months later, the Practice Committee of the RPSGB was advised that the guidance had been revised to include advance supply, but that it had been agreed with the Department of Health and the MHRA not to make any announcement until the patient information leaflet had been revised and a consensus position on the issue of advance supply had been reached among interested stakeholders. The Committee therefore decided to issue the revised guidance, but without reference to advance supply, and so contrary to the revised position of the RPSGB, the Practice Guidance continued to state that 'supply of EHC via the pharmacy in advance of clinical need is not currently recommended'.[25]

Over two years were to pass before the private position of the RPSGB was made public. In December 2006, Marie Stopes International (MSI) and the British Pregnancy Advisory Service (BPAS) announced their support for the advance supply of EHBC. MSI offered a special Emergency Contraception Christmas purse, comprised of a pack of EHBC, two condoms and a Christmas sexual health guide so that women could prepare themselves for the party season,[26] while BPAS ran a 'Just in case' campaign aimed at encouraging women to obtain the drug in advance of need. BPAS Chief Executive, Ann Furedi, claimed:

> It makes sense to keep it in the bathroom cabinet, along with your plasters and paracetamol. You don't wait until you have a headache before buying aspirin, and it makes no sense to wait until you have unprotected sex before you get emergency contraception.[27]

Right on cue, the RPSGB immediately informed the Department of Health that in the light of media attention relating to advance supply, it intended to issue updated recommendations highlighting the fact that

---

[25] Royal Pharmaceutical Society Practice Committee Minutes, 14 September 2004.

[26] Marie Stopes International press release, 'Marie Stopes International to offer special Emergency Contraception Christmas purse for the 2006 festive season', December 2006. However, in February 2007, MSI reported that January had been the busiest ever month for abortion services in its 32 year history. The organisation performed almost 6,000 abortions at its nine UK centres in January, 2007, an increase of 13 per cent on the same month in the previous year. Liz Davies, the director of UK operations at Marie Stopes, put the increase down to 'partying excess and alcohol consumption' over the festive season. Womack S, 'Clinic reports busiest month for abortions', *Daily Telegraph*, 8 February 2007.

[27] British Pregnancy Advisory Service press release, 'Women urged to keep emergency contraceptive pill at home "just in case"', 14 December 2006.

it was not against advance supply in principle. Later that same week, the Society advised pharmacists faced with a request for advance supply of EHBC to use their professional judgment in considering the clinical appropriateness of provision.[28] The Society has, however, not issued any specific guidance in relation to advance provision of EHBC to girls under the age of 16, since supply to this age group remains outside the licensed indications for the over-the-counter version of the product.

[28] Royal Pharmaceutical Society of Great Britain, 'Updated advice on EHC', 18 December 2006 http://www.rpsgb.org/pdfs/pr061218.pdf

3. Primary Care Trusts begin to flex their muscles

Since EHBC has been made available off-prescription, the proportion of women obtaining it from chemists or pharmacies has risen rapidly. In 2005/06, 45 per cent of women aged 16-49 who used EHBC obtained it from a pharmacy, compared with 20 per cent in 2001/02 (Table 1).[1]

Table 1: Where hormonal emergency contraception was obtained
Women aged 16–49 who had used the 'morning after pill' in the year prior to interview, Great Britain

Where obtained	2000/01	2001/02	2002/03	2003/04	2004/05	2005/06
	%	%	%	%	%	%
Own GP or practice nurse	59	43	44	41	33	30
Family planning clinic	33	31	18	21	21	24
Other GP or practice nurse	3	9	5	3	–	1
Hospital Accident & Emergency	3	2	5	5	2	1
Chemist or pharmacy		20	33	27	50	45
A walk-in centre or minor injuries unit		1	0	11	3	4
Other	5	2	4	1	2	1
Base	134	135	129	105	123	67

Percentages add up to more than 100 as respondents could give more than one answer.
Source: ONS, Contraception and Sexual Health, 2005/06

The Department of Health includes the supply of EHBC through pharmacies among the key features of its ten-year strategy for pharmaceutical public health. The provision of 'emergency hormonal contraception under Patient Group Directions' is listed among the 'public health priorities of pharmacies' as a means of reducing the under-18 conception rate and as part of a broader strategy to improve sexual health. According to the document, pharmacy supply of EHBC could have a considerable impact in reducing health inequalities, unwanted conceptions and teenage pregnancy.[2]

---

[1] ONS, Contraception and Sexual Health, 2005/06, Omnibus Survey Report No 30.

[2] Department of Health, Choosing health through pharmacy: A programme for pharmaceutical public health, 2005-2015, April 2005.

Although no figures are available to show how many girls under the age of 16 are obtaining EHBC from pharmacies, the fact that recent years have seen a marked decline in the numbers of underage girls obtaining it from community contraception clinics suggests that growing numbers are accessing it from pharmacies under PGDs (Figure 1).

Figure 1: Prescriptions for EHBC to girls aged under 16 in community contraception clinics: England, 1997/98-2005/06

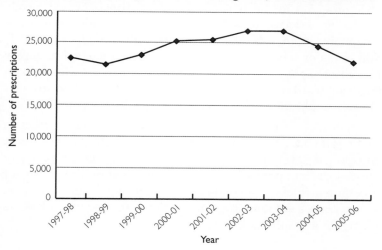

Source: HC Deb (2006-07) 463, written answers, col 1356.

PCTs and under-16s

However, the ease with which growing numbers of girls under the age of 16 are able to obtain EHBC from a variety of sources has not been enough for many Primary Care Trusts (PCTs) and, during 2006, press reports began to appear suggesting that some PCTs were insisting on the provision of EHBC to underage girls as a condition of granting a licence to operate a pharmacy. The supermarket giant, Tesco, found itself being refused a licence to open a pharmacy in some of its superstores simply because of its policy not to supply EHBC to girls under the age of 16.[3] Tesco had taken its principled stance on the issue during 2002 in response to customer concerns.[4]

---

[3] Dawar A, 'Pill for under-16s at Tesco', *Daily Telegraph*, 22 April 2006.
[4] Letter from Tesco, 23 July 2002.

The introduction of the National Health Service (Pharmaceutical Services) Regulations 2005 is being used as a mechanism by a number of PCTs to force new pharmacies to supply EHBC to girls under the age of 16.[5] Under section 12 of the regulations, a PCT only grants an application where it is satisfied it is 'necessary or desirable' to do so in order to secure the adequate provision of pharmaceutical services in a local neighbourhood.[6] This requires PCTs to review the services already provided and to consider whether the package offered by the applicant will enhance provision in the area. If the new pharmacy would merely duplicate existing services, it is likely that an application would be refused. Therefore, in an area where there were already pharmacies offering a full range of services, but where none were prepared to supply EHBC to underage girls, an application which stated a willingness to provide the drug to girls under the age of 16 would be in a much stronger position than an application that indicated an unwillingness to do so.

Where applications are made for a pharmacy licence on premises in an approved retail area, on premises open for at least 100 hours a week, or on premises in a new one-stop primary care centre, the 'necessary or desirable test' does not apply and the PCT may insist on the pharmacy providing certain services as a condition of granting a licence.[7] It is on this basis that Tesco has found itself in conflict with a number of PCTs when applying for a licence to operate in-store pharmacies.

Survey of PCTs

While Tesco had encountered difficulty with at least 13 PCTs,[8] it was unknown precisely how many PCTs were refusing pharmacy licences where applicants declined to provide EHBC to girls under the age of 16. In an attempt to find out how widespread this was, in December 2006 Family Education Trust wrote to all 152 PCTs in England under the provisions of the Freedom of Information Act 2000 with three enquiries:

1. Whether the PCT had issued a PGD permitting the pharmacy supply of EHBC to young women aged under 16;

---

[5] NHS (Pharmaceutical Services) Regulations 2005, http://www.opsi.gov.uk/si/si2005/20050641.htm
[6] HC Deb (2005-06) 447, written answers, col 1542-1543.
[7] NHS (Pharmaceutical Services) Regulations 2005, Section 13.
[8] Burnley, Pendle and Rossendale; North Lincolnshire; North-East Lincolnshire; East Cheshire; Worcestershire; Hampshire and Isle of Wight; South Gloucestershire; Charnwood and North-West Leicestershire; East Sussex; Brighton and Hove; Durham and Chester-le-Street; Erewash; Rugby. Letter from Tesco, 16 June 2006.

2. If a PGD permitting the pharmacy supply of EHBC to young women aged under 16 were in place, whether the PCT insisted on the supply of EHBC to under-16s as a condition of granting a pharmacy licence (under the 'necessary and desirable test' and/or on premises where the test does not apply);

3. Where a PGD permitting the pharmacy supply of EHBC to young women aged under 16 was in place, details of the assessment and evaluation on which the decision to issue it was based were requested.

The responses received revealed that 128 PCTs (84 per cent) had a PGD permitting the supply of EHBC to underage girls (Figure 2). While some PCTs specified a lower age limit of 12, 13, 14 or 15, over half the PGDs supplied made no reference to a lower age threshold.

Figure 2: Does the PCT have a PGD in place permitting the supply of EHBC to under-16s?

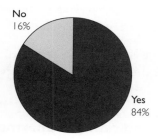

No
16%

Yes
84%

Only a small proportion of PGDs obtained from PCTs referred to the Summary of Product Characteristics (SPC) for the prescription-only product, and with varying degrees of accuracy. For example, while permitting the supply of EHBC to girls under the age of 16 who are able to satisfy specified criteria, the PGD prepared by Cambridgeshire PCT correctly states:

Levonelle 1500 is not recommended in children. Very limited data are available in women under 16 years of age. **Levonelle 1500 is not licensed for women under the age of 16** (emphasis in original).[9]

However, the PGD issued for use by accredited pharmacists in Halton and Warrington makes only an oblique reference to the SPC in the context of stating that EHBC is not to be provided to girls who have not yet reached puberty. Under a section headed 'Exclusion criteria', the PGD states:

Client is pre-pubertal with no established menstrual cycle. Levonelle 1500 is not recommended in children. Limited data are available in young women of childbearing potential aged 14 and under.[10]

Similarly, the Heart of Birmingham Teaching PCT appears to limit the meaning of 'children' to girls under the age of 13. The PGD instructs pharmacists who are approached by girls below that age to refer them to a doctor. The standard referral letter which pharmacists are to issue reads:

I am unable to supply Emergency Hormonal Contraception to this client since she falls outside the Patient Group Direction for the following reason... The client is under 13 years of age (Levonelle 1500 not licensed for children).[11]

Most PGDs supplied made no reference at all to the statement in the SPC that the drug 'is not recommended in children' and that 'very limited data are available' to support its use by under-16s.[12]

Supply of EHBC to under-16s as a condition of a pharmacy licence

Of the 128 PCTs with a PGD, 90 (70 per cent) indicated that they would, under some circumstances, make the supply of EHBC to underage girls a condition of granting a pharmacy licence (Figure 3). Some specifically

[9] Cambridgeshire PCT, Patient Group Direction for Levonorgestrel 1500 microgram tablets by registered pharmacists, October 2007.

[10] Halton PCT and Warrington PCT, Patient Group Direction for the supply and administration of Levonorgestrel 1500 microgram tablets (Levonelle 1500) emergency hormonal contraception (EHC) by accredited pharmacists in Halton and Warrington. Supplied by Warrington PCT, 22 December 2006.

[11] Heart of Birmingham Teaching PCT, Patient Group Directions for the supply of Levonelle 1500 for emergency hormonal contraception, May 2006.

[12] Bayer Schering, Summary of Product Characteristics for Levonelle 1500.
http://www.emc.medicines.org.uk/emc/assets/c/html/displaydoc.asp?documentid=16887

stated they would make a decision based on the need in a given area and would only insist on provision to under-16s where pharmacies were situated in areas where teenage pregnancy rates were high.

Figure 3: Where a PGD is in place, would the PCT ever insist on the supply of EHBC to under-16s as a condition of granting a pharmacy licence?

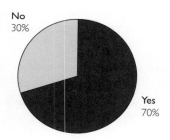

No
30%

Yes
70%

For example, Plymouth PCT stated:

Under certain circumstances of pharmacy application the PCT would insist on a pharmacy providing the Plymouth PCT LES [Local Enhanced Service] for Emergency Hormonal Contraception (in line with the relevant PGD); under other circumstances it would not. The circumstances under which the PCT would insist on this being provided are if: -

• the pharmacy application was exempt from the necessary and desirable test as per the regulations in place at that time as PCTs (as the regulations currently stand) have the right to direct such pharmacies to provide specified enhanced services at the PCT's discretion; and

• the pharmacy was identified as being in a target area for reducing teenage pregnancies as identified and/or ratified by the PCT.[13]

Derbyshire County PCT similarly responded:

The PCT may consider an EHC service is required for exempted criteria applications, although this requirement will differ from locality to locality and may be informed by local need.[14]

Coventry PCT explained that if an established Locally Enhanced Service (LES) were listed in its Pharmaceutical Needs Assessment (PNA), then exempted category pharmacies would have to take part should they be instructed to do so by the PCT. This did not mean, however, that they would automatically be commissioned to provide the service. The PCT went on to relate that:

Problems have occurred when applications have been made for exempted category pharmacies and applicants have said that they would be happy to provide a service listed in the PNA, if so commissioned, but only for some clients and not all those within the inclusion criteria of the PGD.[15]

An example of this would be where a pharmacy was willing to supply EHBC to women aged 16 and over, but unwilling to dispense it to underage girls. Such a response would be unacceptable to Coventry PCT:

The PCT took the view, as have others across England, that this was unacceptable and that we could not have one pharmacy providing the service to one specification and another to a different specification. In the case where we rejected an application on these grounds, the applicant came back with another application and agreed to the specification as already being used across the city.

One point to note, however, is that the PCT would enter negotiations with the pharmacy before directing an LES. The last thing we would want is for a pharmacy to be dragged into a service kicking and screaming even if we could insist by regulation. EHC would not be a service provided from all pharmacies, and we have 83, but in specific localities where teenage pregnancy was an issue. We know from data we have collated ourselves that there is at least one pharmacy in each of these localities who would be willing, and able, to provide the service as per our current specification. If, however, the PCT felt that the only pharmacy

[14] Derbyshire County PCT, 3 January 2007, in relation to South Derbyshire.
[15] Coventry PCT, 9 February 2007.

that could provide the service in a locality was the exempt category pharmacy, then we would have to direct it.[16]

Other PCTs indicated that they would insist on provision of EHBC to girls under the age of 16 as a condition of granting a licence in all pharmacies exempt from the 'necessary or desirable test' irrespective of location. For example, Gloucestershire PCT stated that it currently:

> specifies that all 100 hour pharmacies provide Emergency Hormonal Contraception (EHC) under a Patient Group Direction (PGD). I am also able to confirm that this applies to under 16 year olds.[17]

The rationale for PGDs

When asked for details of the assessment and evaluation leading to the decision to issue a PGD for the supply of EHBC, the vast majority of responses cited high teenage pregnancy rates and the teenage pregnancy strategy. Many PCTs also pointed out that quicker access to EHBC increased the chances of it working. For example, Plymouth PCT stated:

> This scheme was introduced as part of a multi-agency strategy to reduce teenage conceptions and improve young people's sexual health whose aim is to enable young people to make informed choices about their behaviour and to look after their own health.[18]

North Tyneside PCT indicated that teenage conceptions were 'the major driver' behind the PGD, as 'North Tyneside has to achieve a significant reduction to meet government targets',[19] while Luton PCT reported:

> The scheme has been running since December 2002 and the decision to include clients under 16 years of age was due to responses to a questionnaire Luton Pharmacy Development Group sent out to all Luton pharmacies which highlighted that on many occasions supplies of EHC were not made over the counter due to the cost of the product or because the client was under 16.[20]

[16] *ibid.*
[17] Gloucestershire PCT, 31 May 2007.
[18] Plymouth PCT, *op. cit.*
[19] North Tyneside PCT, 21 December 2006.
[20] Luton Teaching PCT, 21 December 2006.

Luton was one of the few PCTs to attempt any justification for insisting that EHBC be supplied to girls under the age of 16 as a condition of granting a pharmacy licence:

> Considering the high priority given to tackling teenage pregnancy and STIs then it would be appropriate to require emergency contraception services to be provided by pharmacy applicants using the exemptions to the controls of entry rules. This requirement should be Luton wide.[68]

Others, like Mid Essex PCT, lamely replied that they were merely following the example of Trusts in other parts of the country:

> It was based on knowledge that it was being undertaken elsewhere and the PCT considered it a positive thing to do.[69]

Portsmouth City PCT is one of the more recent Primary Care Trusts to issue a PGD permitting supply of EHBC to girls under the age of consent in community pharmacies. The Trust's Director of Public Health and Well-being told a local newspaper:

> We have been slower than many other parts of the UK to implement it, as we wanted to be sure of the evidence that it worked before going ahead.[70]

In response to our request for details of the research findings and/or any other factors that had influenced the PCT's decision, the Director referred to several Department of Health strategy and guidance documents before stating that,

> Many experts working locally and nationally in the field of sexual health believe that pregnancy rates and abortion rates would be increasing rapidly without access to emergency contraception.[71]

The Director concluded with an assertion that, 'there is good evidence to show that access to EHC is both effective and welcome'. Once again, we asked Portsmouth City PCT to cite the evidence to substantiate the claim that PGDs permitting pharmacy supply of EHBC would reduce unwanted pregnancy and abortion rates. In reply the Director referred to the 'clinical effectiveness' of the emergency pill, but conceded that:

[21] Luton Teaching PCT, Pharmaceutical Needs Assessment Final Report, March 2006.
[22] Mid Essex PCT, 22 December 2006.
[23] Semke C 'Girls as young as 13 to get free morning-after pill', *The News*, 24 April 2007. http://www.portsmouth.co.uk/news?articleid=2725195
[24] Letter from Portsmouth City PCT, 25 May 2007.

Whether taking this step will actually reduce unwanted pregnancies (whether specifically just in teenagers or in all age groups) and/or reduce abortions remains to be seen.[25]

Significantly not a single PCT has made any attempt to refer to research evidence linking easy access to EHBC with a reduction in teenage pregnancy rates, suggesting that the policies being pursued by the majority of PCTs in this regard may be based, at best, on blind desperation and, at worst, on ideology, rather than on any firm evidence.

[25] Letter from Portsmouth City PCT, 7 October 2007.

4. The evidence base

As we have seen, the government, health agencies and sex educators have expressed tremendous confidence in the ability of EHBC to reduce the rate of unwanted pregnancies. In 1992, American researchers James Trussell from the Office of Population Research at Princeton University and Felicia Stewart from Planned Parenthood of Sacramento Valley calculated that the widespread use of emergency contraception could prevent 1.7 million unintended pregnancies and 0.8 million abortions each year in the USA alone.[1]

Now adjunct professor and co-director of the Center for Reproductive Health Research & Policy at the University of California in San Francisco, Felicia Stewart has more recently claimed that wider access to EHBC is 'perhaps the single most promising avenue for reducing this country's high rates of unintended pregnancy and abortion'.[2]

In the UK, pharmacy supply of the drug has been hailed as a way of making it more readily available to a wider section of the population and a key strand in implementing the government's teenage pregnancy strategy. For example, the RPSGB Expert Advisory Group report referred to in chapter 2 confidently asserted that:

> Pharmacy supply of EHC offers the potential to increase access to the method and thus reduce unwanted pregnancies… EHC…leads to a reduction in the number of unplanned pregnancies and hence the number of likely abortions.[3]

This claim is followed by a reminder that 'the government's target is to halve the pregnancy rate in women aged under 18 by 2010', suggesting that the teenage pregnancy strategy was a prime driver behind pharmacy supply.

But is there any evidence that removing barriers to obtaining EHBC leads to a reduction in rates of unwanted pregnancies and abortions?

---

[1] Trussell J, Stewart F, 'The effectiveness of postcoital contraception', Family Planning Perspectives 1992;24:261–264, cited by Cheng L, Gülmezoglu AM, Van Oel CJ, Piaggio G, Ezcurra E, Van Look PFA, 'Interventions for emergency contraception', *Cochrane Database of Systematic Reviews* 2004, Issue 3.

[2] Quoted in Boonstra H, 'Emergency Contraception: Steps Being Taken to Improve Access', The Guttmacher Report on Public Policy, December 2002, Volume 5, Number 5.

[3] RPSGB Expert Advisory Group report on Emergency Hormonal Contraception, 'Advice on best practice in the supply of Emergency Hormonal Contraception as a Pharmacy medicine', September 2000.

In particular, is there any evidence to demonstrate that the confidential provision of EHBC to underage girls in pharmacies, schools and contraceptive clinics is fulfilling expectations?

PCTs may not have been able to cite data in support of any correlation between the existence of PGDs permitting the supply of EHBC to girls under the age of 16 and areas that have witnessed the greatest reductions in under-16 conception rates, but is there any other evidence to show the effectiveness or otherwise of EHBC to help meet the objectives of the teenage pregnancy strategy?

EHBC and abortion rates

According to an editorial published in the *British Medical Journal* (BMJ) in September 2006, growing use of EHBC has failed to reduce the number of women requesting an abortion in the UK. Abortion rates have continued to rise despite the fact that EHBC is currently being prescribed on around 0.5 million occasions by GPs and family planning clinics in England (Figure 1). In addition, survey data suggest that around 45 per cent of women who take the emergency pill obtain it without prescription from a pharmacy and a further five per cent obtain prescriptions from hospital accident and emergency departments and walk-in centres or minor injuries units.

In her *BMJ* editorial, Professor Anna Glasier, the Director of Family Planning and Well Woman Services at Lothian Primary Care NHS Trust noted that:

> despite the clear increase in the use of emergency contraception, abortion rates have not fallen in the UK. They have risen from 11 per 1000 women aged 15-44 in 1984 (136,388 abortions) to 17.8 per 1000 in 2004 (185,400 abortions). Similarly, increased use of emergency contraception in Sweden has not been associated with a reduction in abortion rates.[4]

During 2006, there was a four per cent increase in the number of abortions performed on women resident in England and Wales over the previous year, taking the total to 193,737 (a rate of 18.3 per 1,000).

---

[4] Glasier A, 'Emergency contraception: Is it worth all the fuss?' *BMJ*, vol 333, 16 September 2006.

Figure 1: Number of abortions performed on women resident in England and Wales, 1968-2006

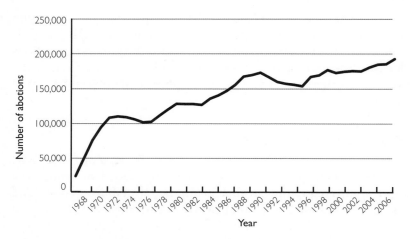

Source: Department of Health, Abortion Statistics, England and Wales: 2006

Professor Glasier, who, during the past five years, has received grants from Schering Health (the company which markets EHBC in the UK) for running educational programmes, points to evidence which suggests that EHBC may not be the solution to rising abortion rates that it has been made out to be. She concedes that the experimental evidence for the effectiveness of EHBC is 'disappointing' and refers to three studies which found that while advance supply of EHBC increased use of the drug, it had no measurable effect on pregnancy or abortion rates.

The proportion of women who seek an abortion having previously taken EHBC has increased from one per cent in 1984, to six per cent in 1996 and 12 per cent in 2002. Professor Glasier concludes: 'If you are looking for an intervention that will reduce abortion rates, emergency contraception may not be the solution.'

The North Carolina systematic review

Professor Glasier's editorial was followed in January 2007 by a study even more devastating to the proponents of easy and widespread access to EHBC. A team of researchers from North Carolina published a systematic review of data on the effects of increased access to EHBC and concluded that there is no evidence to show that increased access has reduced either abortion rates or unintended pregnancy rates.[5] The review of 23 studies from 10 countries published between 1998 and 2006 noted that while there were differences in study design, the primary findings consistently showed no significant differences in unintended pregnancy or abortion rates between women with increased access to the emergency pill and control groups. This was despite the fact that most of the studies showed a substantially higher proportion of women in the intervention group used EHBC than in the control group, and several studies suggested that the intervention also increased the promptness with which emergency pills were taken.

The researchers concluded that while there is now a substantial body of research demonstrating that greater access to EHBC increases its use:

> To date, no study has shown that increased access to this method reduces unintended pregnancy or abortion rates on a population level. The specific interventions varied among the studies, and the quality of some of the studies was poor. Nevertheless, the consistency of their primary findings is hard to ignore.[6]

This conclusion is all the more remarkable bearing in mind the fact that the researchers are themselves fully supportive of EHBC provision in pharmacies. Nevertheless, the weight of the evidence compels them to acknowledge that, 'previous expectations that improved access could produce a direct, substantial impact on a population level may have been overly optimistic'.

The Cochrane review of advance supply

A review of eight studies from the United States, Hong Kong, China and India similarly found that advance provision of EHBC does not lead to a

---

[5] Raymond E G, Trussell, J, Polis C B, 'Population Effect of Increased Access to Emergency Contraceptive Pill', *Obstetrics and Gynecology*, Vol 109, No 1, January 2007.
[6] *ibid*

reduction in unintended pregnancy rates. The studies followed a combined total of over 6,000 women and concluded that while EHBC use was significantly higher in the advance provision group in five studies, the likelihood of pregnancy was just the same regardless of whether or not women had the emergency pill on hand.[7]

The authors of the review published in *The Cochrane Library* remain positive about making EHBC widely and easily accessible. 'Women should have easy access to emergency contraception because it can decrease the chance of pregnancy,' they write. However, they note that:

> Existing data shows that providing women with emergency contraception in advance of need does not reduce unintended pregnancy on a population level... [C]urrent data on advance provision of emergency contraception indicates that tested interventions will not reduce overall unintended pregnancy rates.

[7] Polis C B, Schaffer K, Blanchard K, Glasier A, Harper C C, Grimes D A, 'Advance provision of emergency contraception for pregnancy prevention (full review)', Cochrane Database of Systematic Reviews 2007, Issue 2.

5. Why is emergency hormonal birth control failing?

The evidence that EHBC is not achieving the predicted reduction in unwanted pregnancy and abortion rates is proving an embarrassment to its most enthusiastic advocates. Those who are investing time, money and effort in schemes to make EHBC more readily available to underage girls have tended to react defensively to the international research findings. They are unable to deny the facts, but remain unwilling to review their policies in line with the evidence. So, for example, North Tyneside PCT acknowledges:

> There is no study that is conclusive regarding the use of Emergency Hormonal contraception (EHC) in young people as a strategy to reduce unwanted teenage conception.[1]

Yet despite the absence of any evidence in support of the hypothesis that EHBC will reduce teenage conception rates, North Tyneside presses on with making it available free of charge to underage girls in the hope that it will help meet the government's targets. Its protocol for provision of EHBC confidently states:

> North Tyneside PCT will need to achieve a 55 per cent reduction in teenage pregnancies to meet the teenage conception rate reduction by 2010. The cost of buying POEC [progesterone-only emergency contraception] (£25 per course) excludes many teenage girls from accessing POEC via the community pharmacy. The product licence for over the counter sale further restricts access of this target group, as sales are restricted to those 16 years of age or over.

> This service will reduce the barriers to access to POEC and contribute to a reduction in teenage pregnancies and unwanted pregnancies.[2]

---

[1] Letter from North Tyneside PCT, 13 March 2007.
[2] North Tyneside PCT, Service Level Agreement 2006/08, 'Supply of progestogen only emergency contraception (POEC) – Plan B'.

The fact that on the PCT's own admission there is no evidence that easy access to EHBC reduces teenage conceptions does not prevent it from making assertions that amount to no more than wishful thinking.

When pressed to explain why it is investing in making EHBC available free of charge in some community pharmacies when studies consistently show that easier access is reducing neither abortion nor unplanned pregnancy rates, North Tyneside suggests that without its strategy the situation would be worse than it is currently:

> Where a study demonstrates that teenage pregnancy rates have not declined in an area where free EHC has been implemented, it could be suggested that teenage pregnancy rates could otherwise have been much higher if not implemented.[3]

There is a superficial logic to the PCT's argument at this point. After all, if EHBC works at all – and the evidence suggests that it does have some effectiveness – it stands to reason that it does prevent at least some unwanted pregnancies from developing and thus prevents at least some abortions. Without it, those pregnancies would continue to develop and result in either live births or abortions. The argument then continues: even if EHBC has not made the major inroads into reducing teenage conception rates that its proponents had hoped for, surely it must have brought some benefit even if only in terms of damage limitation. However, this argument only holds if it can be demonstrated that free and easy access to contraception and to EHBC does not adversely affect the sexual behaviour of young people.

Ignorance is not the problem

The government's teenage pregnancy strategy is based on the assumption that young people lack accurate knowledge about contraception and EHBC.[4] Hence the emphasis on sex education, information services and increased availability of contraceptives and emergency pills. But there is growing evidence that this approach does not address the real issues and may prove counterproductive.

---

[3] Letter from North Tyneside PCT, *op. cit.*

[4] Social Exclusion Unit. *Teenage Pregnancy*, London: HMSO, 1999.

Over the past two decades there has been an expansion of sex education programmes in schools, promoting a 'safer sex' message. There has also been a considerable rise in the number of young people attending community contraception clinics in England. The number of first attendances by girls under the age of 16 rose from 18,000 to 83,000 between 1989-90 and 2005-06, while attendances by women overall remained the same (Figure 1).[5] Over a period of less than two decades, the proportion of underage girls attending community contraception clinics has risen from less than two per cent to nearly seven per cent of all attendances. During 2005-06, it is estimated that nearly nine per cent of resident females aged 13-15 attended community contraception clinics in England.[6]

Figure 1: First attendances by girls under 16 at community contraception clinics: England, 1989/90-2005/06

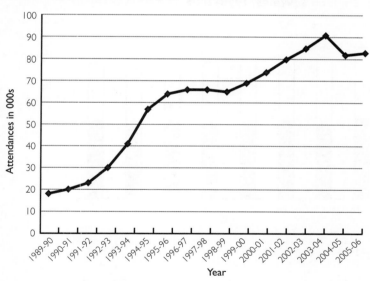

Source: NHS Contraceptive Services, England

[5] Department of Health. *NHS Contraceptive Services, England.*
[6] *ibid.*

Throughout the 1990s, prescriptions for EHBC issued to girls under the age of 16 in community contraception clinics in England increased dramatically and, by 1999/00, represented 10 per cent of prescriptions in that setting. While the numbers of prescriptions for EHBC in community contraception clinics have fallen in recent years due to increased availability in pharmacies, the proportion of prescriptions to girls under the age of 16 continued to rise to 13 per cent of prescriptions in that setting.[7]

Increased access to sexual health advice and contraception, including provision of EHBC, has made no appreciable difference to the recorded conception rates among underage girls, leading either to maternities or to abortions (Figure 2).[8]

Figure 2: Rate of under-16 conceptions and outcomes: England & Wales, 1998-2005

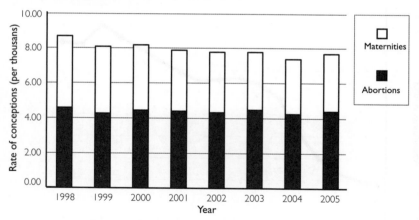

Source: *Teenage Pregnancy Unit*

A study of 240 teenagers who became pregnant found that 93 per cent had seen a health professional at least once during the previous year, and 71 per cent had discussed contraception. The researchers concluded that:

[7] *ibid*

[8] Teenage Pregnancy Unit, *Teenage Conception Statistics for England*, 1998-2005, London: 2007.

- Most teenagers who become pregnant do access general practice in the year before pregnancy, suggesting that potential barriers to care are less than often supposed.

- Teenagers who become pregnant have higher consultation rates than their age-matched peers, and most of the difference is owing to consultation for contraception.

- Teenagers whose pregnancies end in termination are more likely to have received emergency contraception.[9]

The impact of contraception on teenage sexual behaviour

In an article published in the *Journal of Health Economics*, Professor David Paton of Nottingham University Business School examined whether improved family planning services for under-16s were likely to contribute to achieving the aim of reducing underage conceptions. He suggested that the ready availability of contraception might have an impact on the sexual behaviour of young people such that some girls might become sexually active who would not otherwise have done so. Professor Paton tested his hypothesis using figures for attendances at family planning clinics combined with under-16 conception and abortion rates. In particular, he considered the impact of the December 1984 Court of Appeal ruling in the case of Victoria Gillick on under-16 conception rates.[10]

When the Court of Appeal ruled in Mrs Gillick's favour that contraceptive advice should not be given to girls under the age of 16 without parental consent, the sex education and contraception industries predicted the ruling would lead to a marked rise in underage conception rates. However, Professor Paton noted that while attendances by under-16s at family planning clinics decreased by over 30 per cent in the months before the Court of Appeal ruling was overturned in the House of Lords in October 1985, the under-16 conception rate remained unchanged (Figure 3). After the law lords' ruling had lifted the restrictions on contraceptive provision to under-16s it was some time before under-16 family planning attendances returned to previous levels. Yet during the year immediately

[9] Churchill D, Allen J, Pringle M, Hippisley.Cox J, Ebdon D, Macpherson M et al. 'Consultation patterns and provision of contraception in general practice before teenage pregnancy', *BMJ* 2000; 321:486-489.
[10] Paton, D., 'The economics of family planning and underage conceptions', *Journal of Health Economics* 21 (2002) 207-225.

following the judgment in the House of Lords, under-16 conception rates rose by just 0.01 per cent. Professor Paton found no evidence that the Court of Appeal ruling in favour of Mrs Gillick led to an increase in either underage conception or abortion rates.

Figure 3: Rates of under-16 conceptions and attendances at family planning clinics, England 1980-1990

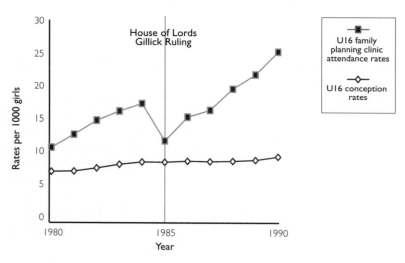

Sources: Teenage Pregnancy Unit and NHS, Contraceptive Services, England, various years

Is EHBC proving counterproductive?

In a subsequent paper published in the *Sex Education* journal, Professor Paton took account of the increased availability of EHBC to girls under the age of 16 but found that the expansion of family planning services to young people under the age of consent was still not showing any association with reduced conception rates notwithstanding the promotion of the emergency pill.[11] Other economists have suggested that the availability of contraception and EHBC 'weakens a woman's bargaining power' and leads to an increase in rates of sexual activity.[12] For many girls the fear of pregnancy serves as a restraint to sexual activity. For some this restraint is overcome by contraceptive provision, while others, conscious of the fact that a large proportion of teenage pregnancies occur as a result of contraceptive failure, are reluctant to take the risk. However, the ready availability of EHBC further reduces the perceived risk of pregnancy and removes one of the major restraints to underage sexual activity.

According to Professor Paton, the fact that increased family planning services for young people are not reducing teenage conception rates and may be contributing to a rise in teenage sexually transmitted infection (STI) rates suggests that the provision of contraception and EHBC may be adversely affecting the sexual behaviour of a significant number of young people.

While Professor Paton surrounds his findings in relation to STIs with several caveats, he urges policy makers to consider the possibility that the introduction of a measure aimed at a specific outcome might carry with it unintended consequences that negate its effectiveness and do more harm than good. He writes:

> In the case in question, there is at least some evidence that some measures aimed at reducing adolescent pregnancy rates induced changes in teenage behaviour that were large enough not only to negate the intended impact on pregnancy rates, but also to have a possible adverse impact on another important area of adolescent sexual health—STIs.[13]

In a separate study published in *Health Economics*, Professor Paton and Dr Sourafel Girma focussed on the impact of over-the-counter provision of EHBC on teenage conceptions, but again found no evidence that it was contributing to lower teenage pregnancy rates.[14] While recent years have seen a massive increase in the number of PCTs offering free provision of EHBC to girls under the age of 16, areas with PGDs permitting pharmacy supply of EHBC to underage girls have not seen greater reductions in conception rates than areas without such provision (Figure 4).

[11] Paton D, 'Random behaviour or rational choice? Family planning, teenage pregnancy and sexually transmitted infections', *Sex Education*, Vol 6, No 3, August 2006.

[12] Akerlof G A, Yellen J L, Katz M L, 'An analysis of out-of-wedlock childbearing in the United States', *Quarterly Journal of Economics*, 111(2) (1996), 277-317, cited by Paton D, *ibid*.

[13] *ibid*

[14] Girma S, Paton D, 'Matching estimates of the impact of over-the-counter emergency birth control on teenage pregnancy', *Health Economics* 15, 2006, 1021-1032.

**Figure 4: Under-16 conception rates and
Pharmacy EHBC schemes, England 1995-2005**

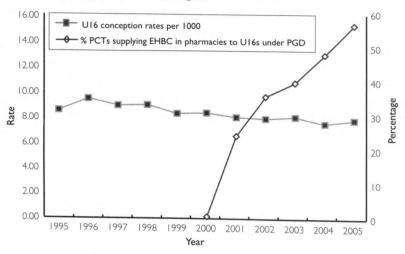

Source: Girma and Paton, Health Economics 2006.

The evidence is mounting that the confidence placed in targeted family planning services for young people combined with promotion of EHBC to make a positive and significant impact on teenage conception rates and unwanted pregnancies has been misplaced. Rather than promoting the sexual health of young people, the perceived reduction in risk afforded by contraception and EHBC appears to be providing some adolescents with an incentive to become sexually active. When introducing measures aimed at reducing teenage conception rates, it is of vital importance to consider the impact of those measures on the behaviour of young people themselves. There is emerging evidence that increased provision of EHBC to underage girls is proving counterproductive and carries with it serious health risks and adverse social consequences.

6. The risks of supplying the emergency pill to underage girls

It is increasingly difficult to understand how PCTs justify investing public funds in making EHBC more easily accessible to teenagers when there is no evidence to support the idea that making emergency pills freely available to underage girls in local pharmacies will contribute to a reduction in teenage pregnancy rates. Indeed, there is evidence that such initiatives may make matters worse by encouraging some girls to become sexually active when they might not otherwise have done so. It is to be feared that in their misplaced reliance on EHBC to reduce teenage conception rates, many health professionals have become blinded to the health risks and adverse social consequences that flow from making contraception and emergency birth control available to girls under the age of consent.

The risk of sexually transmitted infections

Although the Social Exclusion Unit's report on teenage pregnancy warns that a single act of unprotected sex with an infected partner exposes teenage women to a risk of acquiring HIV (one per cent), genital herpes (30 per cent), or gonorrhoea (50 per cent),[1] making EHBC more widely available will do nothing to halt the alarming increase in the incidence of STIs. Indeed, as we have seen, there are concerns that the ready availability of EHBC may lead to an increase in promiscuous behaviour among young people and contribute to a further rise in STI rates.

An article published in *The Lancet* notes that the introduction of a safety device is frequently accompanied by an increase in risk-taking which may cancel out the intended benefit. In some cases, the risk may be transferred from one group of people to another. So, for example, legislation requiring the use of seat-belts in cars was followed by a rise in the rate of

---

[1] Social Exclusion Unit. *Teenage Pregnancy*, London: HMSO, 1999.

deaths among pedestrians, cyclists and rear-seat passengers not wearing a seat-belt, as drivers had been lulled into a false sense of complacency. The authors argue that there is a parallel to be drawn between the use of seat-belts and the more recent rise in the use of condoms to reduce the risk of HIV infection. They refer to evidence that suggests that increased condom usage has been accompanied by a rise in promiscuous behaviour, carrying a high risk of infection.[2]

There is also emerging evidence which suggests that the development of drug therapies to prolong the lives of men infected with HIV has led to increased risk-taking among homosexuals.[3]

A similar trend may be anticipated as a result of the wider availability and promotion of EHBC. While it may reduce the risk of an unwanted pregnancy, it also has the potential to encourage a more casual attitude to sex and expose young people to increased risk of STIs.

Between 1996 and 2005, the total number of diagnoses of STIs made at genitourinary medicine (GUM) clinics increased by 60 per cent and the total workload rose by 268 per cent. In 2005 there were 790,443 diagnoses made and 1,841,886 attendances recorded at sexual health clinics.[4] Over the course of the past decade (1996-2005), there have been marked increases in diagnoses of acute STIs. For example, diagnoses of infectious syphilis have risen by 1954 per cent, genital chlamydia infection by 207 per cent, and genital warts, the most frequently diagnosed viral STI in the UK, by 26 per cent.

Rates of STI diagnoses are continuing to rise among young people aged 16-24. In 2005, 16-24 year olds accounted for 39 per cent of all gonorrhoea diagnoses in men and 70 per cent in women, and the highest rates of gonorrhoea were seen in men aged 20-24 and women aged 16-19. Rates of genital chlamydia infection are highest among young, sexually active men and women. In 2005, men aged 16-24 accounted for 57 per cent of all chlamydia cases in men, and young women aged 16-24 made up 75 per cent of all chlamydia diagnoses in women (Figure 1).

[2] Richens J, Imrie J, Copes A, 'Condoms and seat belts: the parallels and the lessons', *Lancet* 2000; 355:400-403.
[3] Goode E, 'With fears fading, more gays spurn old preventive message', *New York Times*, 19 August 2001.
[4] The UK Collaborative Group for HIV and STI Surveillance, *A Complex Picture. HIV and other Sexually Transmitted Infections in the United Kingdom: 2006.* London: Health Protection Agency, Centre for Infections, November 2006.

Figure 1: STI diagnoses among young people (aged 16-24) as a percentage of total diagnoses across all ages, United Kingdom: 2005

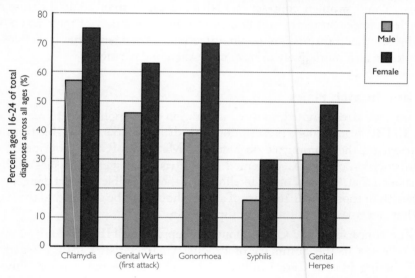

Source: Health Protection Agency, A Complex Picture: HIV and other Sexually Transmitted Infections in the United Kingdom, 2006

Between 2001 and 2005, diagnoses of chlamydia have increased by 81 per cent in men aged 16-19 and 74 per cent in men aged 20-24. Over this same five year period, diagnoses have also increased in women by 47 per cent for those aged 16-19 and by 39 per cent for those aged 20-24. The Health Protection Agency reports that by the end of the third year of the National Chlamydia Screening Programme (NCSP), approximately 180,000 opportunistic screens for chlamydia infection in under 25 year olds had been undertaken outside of GUM settings and detected infection in 10 per cent of young women and 11 per cent of young men. Chlamydia is the biggest cause of ectopic pregnancy and can lead to infertility and cervical cancer.

According to the Alan Guttmacher Institute, there are biological factors which heighten the risk of STIs for sexually active young women in their teens: 'Young women contract [STIs] more easily than adults because they have fewer protective antibodies and the immaturity of their cervix facilitates the transmission of an infection.'[5] Younger sexually active people are also more likely to have more than one partner.[6]

Other health risks

As we have already noted, in its consideration of an application to reclassify EHBC from being a prescription-only drug to make it available from pharmacies, the Committee on Safety of Medicines (CSM) considered that provision of EHBC presented 'special risk management issues' and concluded that, 'because of the likelihood of these possible indirect dangers to health in those under 16 years of age', it should not be supplied to those in that category without medical supervision.[7]

The concerns of the CSM about the supply of EHBC to under-16s are reflected in the Summary of Product Characteristics (SPC) issued by Schering Health Care Limited with regard to the prescription-only product. The SPC states that the drug 'is not recommended in children', adding that 'very limited data are available' to support its use by under-16s.[8] This is qualified somewhat in the SPC for the pharmacy product, which states that it is 'not recommended for use by young women under 16 years of age without medical supervision'.[9]

While the government states that 'medical supervision includes the supply by other health professionals (such as nurses and pharmacists) working to a patient group direction',[10] the Clinical Expert Report generated when the licence holder applied for Pharmacy status was more cautious about the provision of EHBC to girls under the age of 16 in pharmacies. The report considered that it might be difficult for pharmacists to make the necessary assessment of an underage girl requesting EHBC even if a private area were available. It noted that 'doctors have

---

[5] Alan Guttmacher Institute, *Sexually Transmitted Diseases Hamper Development Efforts*, 1998 http://www.agi-usa.org/pubs/ib_std.html

[6] Dawe F, Meltzer H. *Contraception and Sexual Health*, 1999. London: HMSO, 2001.

[7] Committee on Safety of Medicines, Summary of the Committee on Safety and Medicines meeting held on Thursday 23 March 2000.

[8] http://emc.medicines.org.uk/emc/assets/c/html/displaydoc.asp?documentid=16887

[9] http://emc.medicines.org.uk/emc/assets/c/html/displaydoc.asp?documentid=15227

[10] HC Deb (2001-02) 378, written answers, col 964.

been trained to deal with this aspect of prescribing and are more likely to know the girl's family' and concluded that:

> It may be in the best interests of these young patients to have a consultation with a doctor as there are often complex health and social issues which a pharmacist may not be adequately trained (or have the appropriate facilities) to deal with.[11]

A *Daily Mail* investigation conducted shortly after EHBC was licensed as a Pharmacy medicine for over-16s found that it was possible for girls under that age to purchase the drug with relative ease. Fifteen year-old Charlotte Jacks experienced no difficulty in obtaining EHBC from six out of the seven South London pharmacies she visited. Dr George Rae, the chairman of the British Medical Association's prescribing committee commented:

> The experience of this girl raises serious questions about the need for pharmacists and GPs to have a proper medical record for each person requesting this medication.[12]

> The intent of getting teenage pregnancy down is a good one, but unless you have a central electronic record and the pharmacist and school nurse share this information with the GP, there is a serious risk of fragmentation. As more people get involved in prescribing we must ensure there is proper co-ordination.[13]

The following issues are particularly pertinent in connection with the supply of EHBC to underage girls in pharmacies or other settings where their full medical history is not known:

- The safety of medications can only be determined if health professionals trained to identify side effects follow individuals receiving the drugs over an extended time period because a serious side effect may not be immediately apparent. However, PGDs do not permit a study of this nature to be undertaken;
- There is a lack of scientific data on the long-term effects of EHBC on adolescents, and on its use by females not screened for medical contraindications;

---

[11] Clinical Expert Report, para 7.1 'Age'.

[12] Marsh B, 'The Pill free-for-all', *Daily Mail*, 6 January 2001. In a subsequent parliamentary debate, the health minister Yvette Cooper stated that it was an offence under the Medicines Act 1968 for pharmacists knowingly to supply the Pharmacy product to girls under the age of 16. Prescription Only Medicines (Human Use Amendment (no. 3) Order 2000 (Fifth Standing Committee), 24 January 2001.

[13] Marsh B, 'Morning-after pill free at schools', *Daily Mail*, 8 January 2001.

- While the BPAS leaflet assures readers that, 'Repeat use poses no risk',[14] the maximum safe dose for levonorgestrel has not been determined by scientific study. It is unknown whether there is a maximum safe daily, monthly, or yearly dose. The health risks for those who may use EHBC repeatedly at one time or over a period of years are therefore unknown;

- Adolescents, whose bodies are developing and undergoing rapid hormonal changes, are among those most likely to use EHBC repeatedly. The ability to obtain it in confidence adds to its attraction, but has the effect of making young teenagers more reluctant to seek medical help if complications arise. Underage girls are also less likely to follow the directions for administration. Those particularly anxious about the possibility that they may be pregnant may take more than a single dose, either in the belief that to do so would increase its chances of working, or in an attempt to alleviate the side effect of nausea.

Lessons from America

It is worthy of note that in approving Plan B (the US version of Levonelle One Step) for over-the-counter use in the United States, the Food and Drugs Administration (FDA) has recently given its decision that provision should be restricted to women aged 18 and over.[15]

The Center for Drug Evaluation and Research had previously rejected an application to make Plan B available over the counter to females under the age of 17 on the basis that there was insufficient evidence that EHBC could be used safely by young adolescent women without 'the professional supervision of a practitioner licensed by law to administer the drug'.[16]

That decision was reaffirmed on 26 August 2005, when the Director of the Center for Drug Evaluation and Research found that:

> The data provided support approval for OTC [over the counter] use for women 17 and over, but I am unable to conclude based on the data that women age 16 or less can use OTC Plan B safely and effectively.[17]

---

[14] BPAS, Just in case, December 2006.

[15] Memorandum from Steven Galson, MD, MPH, Director, Center for Drug Evaluation and Research, 24 August 2006, http://www.fda.gov/cder/drug/infopage/planB/memo.pdf

[16] Letter from Steven Galson, MD, MPH, Acting Director, Center for Drug Evaluation and Research, 6 May 2004 http://www.fda.gov/cder/drug/infopage/planB/planB_NALetter.pdf

[17] Memorandum from Steven Galson, MD, MPH, Director, Center for Drug Evaluation and Research, 26 August 2005.

The more recent decision to restrict over-the-counter use of Plan B to women aged 18 and over (rather than to those aged over 17 as previously intimated) was made because it was considered a 'more appropriate cutoff point to best promote and protect the public health'. In the view of Dr Andrew C Von Eschenbach, the Acting Commissioner of the United States Food and Drug Administration, since retail outlets, including pharmacies, were familiar with using 18 as the age restriction for the sale of certain products, it made sense to limit the availability of Plan B to those over the age of 18. Dr Von Eschenbach considered that:

> This approach should minimize the likelihood that younger girls for whom Plan B has not been found safe and effective for non-prescription use will have access to the product without professional supervision. Therefore, this approach should help ensure safe and effective use of the product.[18]

Child protection issues

In the UK, however, there are no such legal restrictions concerning the supply of EHBC to minors and this has given rise to child protection concerns. Some PCTs have issued PGDs without any stated lower age limit, permitting the supply of EHBC to girls of any age, while others do specify a lower age. In North Tyneside, for example, provision is limited to girls aged 13 and above because sexual activity below that age gives rise to child protection concerns. However, it is equally possible that 13-15 year-old girls seeking EHBC may be subject to sexual abuse, and it is also possible that an older girl may obtain emergency birth control on behalf of a girl under the age of 13.

In response to these concerns, North Tyneside simply states that pharmacists must exercise 'professional judgment, a skill used on a daily basis by NHS providers, drawing upon experience and training'. The PCT has not issued any specific guidance to pharmacists on this point, but is content to leave it up to the discretion of the individual:

> Each practitioner will decide how they make those decisions, some may request proof of age, or identity.[19]

---

[18] Memorandum from Dr. Andrew C. Von Eschenbach, Acting Commissioner, United States Food and Drug Administration, 23 August 2006 http://www.fda.gov/cder/drug/infopage/planB/avememo.pdf

[19] Letter from North Tyneside PCT, 13 March 2007.

Such responses are hardly reassuring and reinforce the fact that the easier it becomes to obtain EHBC confidentially and without charge, the more scope there is for the exploitation and abuse of young people.

The messages being conveyed to young people

Making EHBC available to underage girls is contributing to a culture which will have a number of further damaging consequences. Several powerful messages are being conveyed:

(a) There is nothing wrong with engaging in sex at any age.
Provided a condom is used to minimise the risk of pregnancy and/or STIs, the impression is commonly given that there is no real objection to teenage sex outside of marriage. The confidential provision of emergency birth control to girls under the age of 16 is undermining the law on the age of consent and sending out the message that there is nothing wrong with underage sex.

(b) Actions need not have lasting consequences.
While 'safer sex' is encouraged, it is acknowledged that not all will practise it, and among those who do, it may fail. Enter EHBC... All is not lost, because a pill is now readily available which, if taken within 72 hours, has the potential to put any resulting pregnancy to a swift end.

(c) There is a drug to deal with every eventuality.
According to much current thinking, the only thing 'wrong' with teenage sex is that it may leave girls with an unwanted child who may blight their future education and career prospects. Rather than encouraging them to control their own behaviour, they are being directed to a drug which will help control the unwanted consequences of that behaviour.

Over recent years we have witnessed the systematic removal of every restraint which in previous generations served as a disincentive to under-age sexual activity. Sex education in many schools has set out to break down the natural inhibitions of children with regard to sexual conduct; the age of consent is rarely enforced, so young people no longer have any fear of legal proceedings; the ready availability of contraception means that a girl's fear of pregnancy is no longer considered a good enough reason for rejecting her boyfriend's advances; and confidentiality policies mean that a girl need not worry about what her parents would think about her being sexually active, obtaining contraception, being treated for an STI or even having an abortion, because they need not know.

Against such a background, there can be no doubt that the free and confidential provision of EHBC to girls under the age of 16 is further promoting a casual approach to sexual relationships. Young men are now able to put pressure on vulnerable girls to have sex by telling them that if they are worried about getting pregnant, they can always go to a local chemist the following day and get 'the morning-after pill' free of charge. This will inevitably result in more underage sex, more teenage pregnancies, more STIs, and more disjointed families.

In addition to the health risks, the child protection issues and the messages being conveyed by the confidential provision of EHBC to girls under the age of consent, the implications of such initiatives for the role of parents is another major area of concern. The confidentiality policies operated by health authorities strike right at the heart of the relationship between parents and children.

7. Keeping it confidential

In 1985, the House of Lords overturned a Court of Appeal ruling that contraception should not be supplied to girls under the age of 16 without the knowledge and consent of their parents. However, in delivering their judgment, the law lords were insistent that under all normal circumstances the child's parents should be informed and in agreement with the supply of contraceptive treatment to an underage girl. Lord Scarman ruled:

> ...a doctor is only in exceptional circumstances to prescribe contraception to a young person under the age of 16 without the knowledge and consent of a parent... Only in exceptional cases does the guidance contemplate [a doctor] exercising his clinical judgement without the parents' knowledge and consent.[1]

Lord Fraser concurred:

> Nobody doubts, certainly I do not doubt, that in the overwhelming majority of cases the best judges of a child's welfare are his or her parents. Nor do I doubt that any important medical treatment of a child under 16 would normally only be carried out with the parents' approval. That is why it would and should be most unusual for a doctor to advise a child without the knowledge and consent of parents on contraceptive matters.

Many health professionals continue to appeal to the 'Fraser criteria' to defend the confidential provision of contraception to a girl under the age of consent: (i) that she will understand the advice given; (ii) that she cannot be persuaded to tell her parents; (iii) that she is likely to begin or continue in a sexual relationship; (iv) that her physical or mental health may suffer if contraceptive treatment is denied her; and (v) that it is in her best interests.[2] However, few are aware that Lord Fraser added that these criteria:

---

[1] Gillick v West Norfolk and Wisbech Area Health Authority and another - [1985] 3 All ER 402.
[2] For example, according to guidance issued by the Faculty of Family Planning and Reproductive Health Care Clinical Effectiveness Unit: 'The Law Lords' ruling (the Fraser ruling) stated that a clinician may provide contraceptive advice and treatment to a young person under the age of 16 years, without parental consent, provided that he/she has confirmed that the young person is competent and that the Fraser criteria (advice understood, will have or continue to have sex, advised to inform parents, in their best interest) are met.' FFPRHC Guidance (April 2006) Emergency contraception', *Journal of Family Planning and Reproductive Health Care*, 2006, 32(2), 121-128.

ought not to be regarded as a licence for doctors to disregard the wishes of parents on this matter whenever they find it convenient to do so. Any doctor who behaves in such a way would, in my opinion, be failing to discharge his professional responsibilities, and I would expect him to be disciplined by his own professional body accordingly.

In 1985, it was not widely envisaged that two decades later contraception and EHBC would be available to increasing numbers of children in clinics operating on school premises, underage girls would be able to access emergency birth control in local pharmacies, and three-fifths of PCTs would be prepared under some circumstances to insist on underage provision as a condition of granting a pharmacy licence.

Confidentiality and the teenage pregnancy strategy

The Social Exclusion Unit's report on teenage pregnancy, published in 1999, stressed the importance of making contraception available in confidence to young people under the age of consent and ensured that confidentiality was placed at the heart of the teenage pregnancy strategy. The report revealed that the government's action plan included Department of Health funding for 'a national publicity campaign to make young people aware that they have a right to talk to health professionals about sex, relationships and contraception in confidence'.[3]

In July 2004, the Department of Health's revised guidance to health professionals on contraception, sexual and reproductive health services (including abortion) for under-16s continued to place a strong emphasis on 'the duty of confidentiality'. It states that:

All services providing advice and treatment on contraception, sexual and reproductive health should produce an explicit confidentiality policy which...makes clear that young people have the same right to confidentiality as adults.[4]

The guidance goes on to stress that such confidentiality policies 'should be prominently advertised, in partnership with education, youth and community services'. Unless there is 'a risk to the health, safety or

---

[3] Social Exclusion Unit. *Teenage Pregnancy*, London: HMSO, 1999.

[4] Department of Health, 'Best practice guidance for doctors and other health professionals on the provision of advice and treatment to young people under 16 on contraception, sexual and reproductive health', 29 July 2004.

welfare of a young person or others which is so serious as to outweigh the young person's right to privacy', any deliberate breach of confidentiality is to be treated as a serious disciplinary matter.

At no point does the guidance refer to the law on the age of consent. The impression is given throughout that young people are free to make an 'informed choice' about engaging in an unlawful sexual relationship under the age of 16. The only reference to statute appears in a section designed to assure health professionals that:

> the Sexual Offences Act 2003 does not affect the ability of health professionals and others working with young people to provide confidential advice or treatment on contraception, sexual and reproductive health to young people under 16.[5]

Under the terms of the Sexual Offences Act, health professionals, teachers, Connexions Personal Advisers, youth workers, social practitioners, parents and anyone else acting to protect a child, are deemed to be 'not guilty of aiding, abetting or counselling' a sexual offence against a child where they are acting for the purpose of:

- protecting a child from pregnancy or sexually transmitted infection,
- protecting the physical safety of a child, or
- promoting a child's emotional well-being by the giving of advice.[6]

In other words, the confidential provision of contraception to young people under the legal age of consent is justified on the basis that it may help the child to avoid becoming pregnant or contracting an STI. There is perhaps no other area on which the government presents breaking the law as an option and even helps to facilitate lawbreaking, or at least sets out to mitigate the consequences of unlawful conduct.

More recently, the General Medical Council (GMC) has issued guidance on the roles and responsibilities of doctors in relation to children and young people. The guidance advises doctors that, subject to the 'Fraser criteria':

> You can provide contraceptive, abortion and STI advice and treatment, without parental knowledge or consent, to young people under 16.[7]

[5] *ibid.*
[6] Sexual Offences Act 2003, s73.
[7] General Medical Council, *0–18 years: guidance for all doctors*, September 2007, para 70.

Elsewhere it asserts:

A confidential sexual health service is essential for the welfare of children and young people. Concern about confidentiality is the biggest deterrent to young people asking for sexual health advice. That in turn presents dangers to young people's own health and to that of the community, particularly other young people.[8]

Many health authorities and contraceptive clinics have issued their own confidentiality statements to encourage young people of any age to seek advice. One such statement offers the following assurance:

Although strictly speaking, it's illegal for someone to have sex with a girl under 16, we know that maturity does not suddenly arrive on the 16th birthday, and that many young people are mature enough to make their own decisions about their lives.

Things are usually easier for young people if they can discuss their relationships with their parent(s), and parent(s) can be very understanding and supportive. Unfortunately, things are not always like this, and we believe that it is up to clients to decide whether or not to tell anyone at home about their visit here.[9]

It is difficult to imagine such a casual approach being taken to law-breaking in any other area. We have yet to see a notice stating:

Although strictly speaking, it's illegal to drive a car under the age of 17, we know that maturity does not suddenly arrive on the 17th birthday, and that many young people are mature enough to make their own decisions about whether or not to drive.

Confidentiality for under-13s

Some medical bodies and contraception advocacy groups are so committed to the principle of confidentiality that they are prepared to bypass established child protection procedures. For example, a protocol for working with sexually active young people prepared by the London Child

---

[8] *ibid.*, para 64.
[9] Whitton Family Planning Clinic, 'Confidentiality Statement'.

Protection Committee (LCPC) came under fire from the *fpa*, Brook and the British Medical Association (BMA) for undermining the confidentiality that they felt was owed to young people.

The LCPC document insisted that: 'It must always be made clear to children and young people...that the duty of confidentiality is not absolute', and added that, 'All cases of children under the age of 13 years who are believed to be or have been engaged in penetrative sexual activity must be referred to Children's Social Services and the Police as a potential case of rape.'[10]

With regard to sexually active 13-15 year-olds, the LCPC protocol stated that any decision not to make a formal referral to the police should be made by a senior member of staff after establishing that the child was not being abused or exploited and after checking police indices. However, where there were concerns that a sexual relationship presents a risk of harm to a child over the age of 13, the LCPC protocol insisted that 'a referral *must* be made to Children's Social Services and the Police' (emphasis in original). Where the practitioner's assessment does not raise abuse concerns, the agency is encouraged to 'make arrangements for the young person to receive confidential advice and support from appropriate sexual health and other services'.

Vivienne Nathanson, the Head of Ethics at the BMA objected to mandatory reporting of sexual relationships involving children under the age of 13. She held the key issue was to ensure that young people had the confidence to negotiate about whether they wanted to be sexually active, including the ability to negotiate and say no. Asked about the responsibility of doctors towards the parent of an underage child who was engaging in sexual activity, Dr Nathanson insisted:

> It's not to the parents; it's to the child. It's the child who is the patient. And it's in the child's best interests to give that child good advice, to try to make sure that child is not involved in a relationship that is abusive or coercive.... But for the parent's sake, the point is that the doctor is there to look after their child's welfare.[11]

The chief executive of Brook, Jan Barlow, commented that the protocol

---

[10] London Child Protection Committee, 'Working with Sexually Active Young People under the age of 18 – a Pan-London Protocol', April 2005.
[11] BBC Radio 4, *Today*, 30 September 2005.

went 'against everything we believe in'. In a written statement on 'Under-16s and sexual activity', the *fpa* insisted that young people, including those under the age of 13, were entitled to confidentiality when accessing sexual health services and held that it was 'crucial that professionals do not confuse child protection issues with the normal sexual development of young people'.[12] In support of its position, the *fpa* cited a Home Office document stating that:

> Although the age of consent remains at 16, the law is not intended to prosecute mutually agreed teenage sexual activity between two young people of a similar age, unless it involves abuse or exploitation. Young people, including those under 13, will continue to have the right to confidential advice on contraception, condoms, pregnancy and abortion.[13]

In its guidance to doctors on consultations with children from birth to 18, the GMC falls short of advocating mandatory reporting of sexually active children below the age of 13. The guidance states that, 'You should *usually* share information about sexual activity involving children under 13, who are considered in law to be unable to consent' (emphasis added),[14] but since the guidance takes the view that 'the capacity to consent depends more on young people's ability to understand and weigh up options than on age',[15] it leaves the door open to extending the right of confidentiality to sexually active pre-teens.

The Commissioner for Children and Young People has also made it clear that he supports the right of young people to engage in unlawful sexual intercourse well below the age of consent and to obtain contraceptive advice and treatment without the knowledge of their parents. In his first annual report, Sir Al Aynsley-Green maintains that, 'opposing mandatory reporting of sexual activity in under-13s' fulfils the *Every Child Matters* objectives to 'Be healthy' and 'Stay safe'.[16] A response to the pan-London protocol on working with sexually active people under the age of 18 prepared by Professor Carolyn Hamilton of the Children's Legal Centre on behalf of the Children's Commissioner goes further. It suggests that a requirement on professionals to report a young person for

---

[12] FPA, Statement on 'Under-16s and sexual activity', July 2005.
[13] Home Office, 'Working within the Sexual Offences Act 2003', 2004.
[14] General Medical Council, *0-18 years: guidance for all doctors*, op. cit., para 67.
[15] *ibid.*, para 25.
[16] Office of the Children's Commissioner, Annual Report 2005/06, London: TSO, HC1278, July 2006

underage sexual activity 'could be considered an invasion of the young person's right to private life'.[17]

Parents do not appear to feature very prominently in the thinking of the Children's Commissioner's office, nor in the minds of the *fpa*, Brook, and senior figures at the BMA and GMC. There are also grounds to fear that some doctors may be excluding parents and placing children at risk of sexual abuse and exploitation in the name of the right of the child to confidential treatment.

---

[17] Office of the Commissioner for Children, Response to 'Working with sexually active people under the age of 18 – a pan-London protocol'.

8. Who needs parents?

In the course of giving oral evidence before the Joint Committee on Human Rights, the President of the Royal College of Paediatrics and Child Health, Professor David Hall, was asked about the provision of contraception to a 12-year-old girl involved in a sexual relationship with a 22-year-old man. The questioner explained:

> The parents are livid and want the full force of the law brought to bear on that situation. The child herself appears to be consenting and maintaining the position that she is capable of making her own decisions and the law of course says that that relationship, if it is taking place, is statutory rape which has a sentence of life imprisonment as a maximum. If the child in that situation wants contraceptive advice and contraception, how do you we *(sic)* deal with that terribly difficult situation?

Professor Hall responded:

> The advice that GPs receive...would be that as far as the young person herself is concerned you would have to make a judgment as her doctor about the right course of action. If your judgment was that she was making a mature and considered decision in coming to consult you and was asking for contraceptive advice, I think most doctors would provide that advice and treat that in confidence. If their judgment was that this girl was being manipulated and used then the terms used include 'some secrets are too big to keep'. That might be the sort of language you would use to someone you treat as a child. In the case you describe I suspect most people would feel that as far as their behaviour as a doctor was concerned, they would probably give her the advice that she was requesting because they would consider her very competent by the very act of having come to seek advice on contraception and they would consider that was how she was behaving. They would probably then ring their Medical Defence Union and say, 'Help, have I done the right thing?' I think that is probably what most of them would do.[1]

---

[1] Joint Committee on Human Rights, Twenty-second Report of Session 2001-02, The Case for a Human Rights Commission: Interim Report, HL Paper 160, HC 1142, Ev 60.

If Professor Hall is correct in his assessment of current GP practice, it is to be feared we have lost sight of the protective provisions of the legal age of consent to sexual intercourse and the protective instincts of the child's parents. We have also moved a long way from the judgment of the law lords in *Gillick v West Norfolk and Wisbech Area Health Authority*, when Lord Fraser ruled that, 'any important medical treatment of a child under 16 would normally only be carried out with the parents' approval' and that it should therefore be 'most unusual for a doctor to advise a child without the knowledge and consent' of parents on contraceptive matters'.[2]

During the course of the two decades since the Gillick ruling, the exception has become the norm. Girls under the age of 16 are now routinely supplied with contraception, EHBC and even abortions without the knowledge or consent of their parents. Not content with making EHBC freely available to girls under the age of 16 at community contraception clinics and pharmacies in many parts of the country, health and education bodies, in conjunction with contraception advocates, are encouraging school heads and governing bodies to make contraception and EHBC available on school premises. The Director of Communications for the British Pregnancy Advisory Service suggests:

> [F]or emergency contraception to be used effectively by teenagers, it needs to be provided conveniently, confidentially and cheaply (preferably free of charge altogether)...Teenagers are more likely to benefit from projects that take free contraceptive services into their schools...[3]

School nurses

In March 2006, the government issued fresh guidance for headteachers, teachers, support staff and governors to help them expand or develop a school nursing service, including the provision of confidential contraceptive and abortion advice to underage pupils. According to the document, *Looking for a School Nurse?* the provision of contraceptive advice, together with 'emergency contraception' and pregnancy testing on school premises, will prevent teenage pregnancies and reduce the rates of sexually transmitted infections.[4]

---

[2] Gillick v West Norfolk and Wisbech Area Health Authority and another - [1985] 3 All ER 402.
[3] Furedi A. 'Pharmacy sale of emergency contraception', *Childright* 175, April 2001.
[4] Department of Health, *Looking for a School Nurse?* March 2006,
http://www.dh.gov.uk/assetRoot/04/13/21/96/04132196.pdf

Alongside the guidance to schools, the government has also published the *School Nurse: Practice Development Resource Pack*, offering best practice guidance to school nurses and public health officials. The guidance states that, 'school nurses can raise sexual health and relationship issues with young people and make sure they have access to the kind of information and services they need.' As part of 'best practice', school nurses are encouraged to:

- Provide and promote confidential drop-ins at school and community venues, ensuring they are linked to wider primary health care, family planning and genitourinary medicine (GUM) services. Consider the use of new technologies such as texting or e-mail to improve access.

- Ensure that sex and relationship education [SRE] programmes and services meet the needs of ethnic minority, disabled, bisexual, transgender, gay and lesbian young people. Confront discrimination and challenge prejudice such as homophobia.

- Support young women to access services to make timely choices about emergency contraception, pregnancy or abortion.

- Clarify the purpose and boundary of your role within SRE, ensure it is clear to young people, use ground rules in sessions and remind young people where they can access confidential support and information.[5]

More recently, Ofsted has added its voice in support of the confidential provision of EHBC on school premises. Its report *Time for change? Personal, social and health education* stated that:

School nurses can…provide a valuable service, particularly in terms of providing emergency hormonal contraception and advising on other forms of contraception.[6]

When Ofsted were asked how they could say this when research consistently showed that supplying EHBC was not making the slightest difference to teenage pregnancy and abortion rates, they lamely replied that pupils said they appreciated it:

---

[5] Department of Health, *School Nurse: Practice Development Resource Pack*, March 2006.
  http://www.dh.gov.uk/assetRoot/04/13/20/70/04132070.pdf
[6] Ofsted, *Time for change? Personal, social and health education*, April 2007.

The basis on which the report states that school nurses can also provide a valuable service, particularly in terms of providing emergency hormonal contraception, is again based on our discussions with students in secondary schools where students said they found services provided by school nurses useful and helpful. We made no claim that they reduce teenage pregnancy or abortion rates.[7]

Apparently, in the view of the Office for Standards in Education, if pupils value being able to get contraception and emergency pills from the school nurse in strict confidence without Mum and Dad knowing, that makes it a valuable service, irrespective of whether it contributes to a reduction in teenage pregnancy and abortion rates.

Subsequent correspondence confirmed that Ofsted had not taken any account of research showing that access to EHBC had not resulted in a reduction in unwanted pregnancy or abortion rates, 'as this was a report based, in the main, on first-hand evidence from inspectors' visits to schools'.[8]

It does not bode well for children when the body responsible for improving standards in schools is blindly following the dictates of the sex education establishment and the Teenage Pregnancy Unit, and when it cannot tell the difference between what children say they value and what is truly valuable.

Clinics in schools

As recently as 2001, it was relatively rare for contraception and EHBC to be supplied to pupils on school premises and the government appeared wary of openly supporting such initiatives. In response to a parliamentary question, health minister Jacqui Smith stated:

> We would not normally expect school nurses to issue contraception or emergency contraception. In the few cases where school nurses are dispensing contraception, this should be made clear in the school's sex and relationships education policy which has to be agreed with parents. These arrangements should not proceed until parents have been consulted.[9]

[7] Letter from Ofsted, 18 April 2007.
[8] Letter from Ofsted, 26 June 2007.
[9] HC Deb (2001-02) 362, written answers, col 485.

Now, however, at the instigation of PCTs and with the full encouragement of Ofsted, a growing number of schools are introducing health clinics on school premises with a particular emphasis on offering contraceptive advice and supplying contraception and EHBC. These clinics are known by different names in different parts of the country. For example, in Oxfordshire, they are known as Bodyzone, while in some parts of Devon and Cornwall they operate under the name of TIC-TAC (Teenage Information Centre, Teenage Advice Centre). Lutterworth Grammar School and Community College, which hit the headlines in April 2007 for distributing EHBC to pupils on 345 occasions over a period of four years offers a student advisory service known as 'Strictly Confidential'.

Children attending a Bodyzone clinic are issued with a welcome form which assures them that 'this is a completely CONFIDENTIAL service...your school/college are not allowed to ask why you are attending Bodyzone' (emphasis in original). The first option on the form is for children to ask for 'The Sexual Health Nurse (for contraception, pregnancy tests, supplies and advice)'. The Bodyzone project pack explains that the family planning nurse can '...issue condoms, emergency contraception and repeat supplies of the pill and injectables without a doctor present'.[10] During the first year the scheme operated in Oxfordshire schools, around 140 teenage girls were given EHBC without their parents' prior knowledge.[11]

The guidance of the former Department for Education and Employment (DfEE) on sex and relationship education emphasises that parents are the key people in teaching their children about sex and relationships and that '[s]chools should always work in partnership with parents, consulting them regularly on the content of sex and relationship education programmes'.[12]

However, in many parts of the country, the guidance on sex and relationships education with its emphasis on parental responsibility is being by-passed by projects operated by health authorities in the context of the local school. Education legislation is similarly being circumvented. Under the Education Act 1993, parents have an unconditional right to withdraw their children from any sex education in school with the exception of 'biological aspects' required by the National Curriculum. However, since

---

[10] Bodyzone Information Pack 2.

[11] Owen V, 'Clinics give pill to 140 schoolgirls', *Oxford Times*, 24 August 2001.

[12] Department for Education & Employment, 'Sex and Relationship Education Guidance', London: HMSO July 2000.

Bodyzone and other similar schemes operate outside the school curriculum as a service of the health authority, they are not subject to primary education law nor covered by the DfEE guidance.

With regard to the availability of EHBC in a school setting, the government's position is that:

> [W]here a school nurse provides emergency contraception she works within the same legal framework and government guidance as other health professionals providing contraception to under-16s. They must always encourage the young person to involve her parents, but the nurses' professional code states that, if the girl refuses, confidentiality must be maintained unless there are serious child protection issues.[13]

Asked who would take responsibility in the event of a pupil under the age of 16 suffering an adverse reaction as a direct consequence of being supplied with EHBC on school premises, whether with or without the sanction of the governing body, the government has stated that the school nurse would be accountable, but would have vicarious liability protection with the NHS or Primary Care Trust that employed her, provided she acted with their consent. According to the education minister, Beverley Hughes, the responsibility of school governors extends no further than ensuring that parents are adequately consulted and ensuring that a protocol exists with the PCT/trust that makes clear which services will be delivered by PCT/trust staff working on the school site.[14]

TIC-TAC

Paignton Community and Sports College has been in the forefront of the promotion of confidential school-based provision of contraception and EHBC. The Principal, Jane English, is a member of the Independent Advisory Group on Teenage Pregnancy and a keen advocate of family planning services in schools. In the College prospectus for 2006, she writes:

> TIC-TAC (Teenage Information Centre/Teenage Advice Centre) is available to students every lunchtime... The Centre has received praise from the NHS,

---

[13] HL Deb (2000-01) 621, col.560.
[14] HC Deb (2005-06) 447, col 533.

OFSTED and the Government's Select Committee... The College delivers Sex and Relationships Education and the TIC-TAC Centre plays a vital supplementary role in this programme. Following these lessons the number of pupils attending the Centre increases as young people go along to ask questions they felt too shy to ask in front of their classmates.

Over the past five years the College has, through gaining Beacon Status and Teenage Pregnancy Unit Conferences, shared its good practice around the country and we are delighted that more schools are now looking to work in collaboration with Health Authorities.

As Principal of the College I consider myself very fortunate to have a Governing Body who, mindful of the issues, had the foresight to be pioneering. TIC-TAC is very successful, every school should have one.[15]

However, not all share the Principal's enthusiasm for the confidential service offered at Paignton Community and Sports College. Kerry Neal, the mother of 14 year-old Kizzy, a pupil at the College, who gave birth to a child in May 2007, has been particularly critical. She considers that:

> [T]he ease of access to contraception for these young people, including extremely aggressive forms such as the morning-after-pill, seems to be making these young and impressionable minds complacent about their whole attitude towards acceptable sexual behaviour.[16]

While acknowledging the social problems associated with teenage pregnancy, she is horrified that EHBC is being given to pupils in her own daughter's situation, often without the knowledge and consent of their parents. She also expresses concern at the pressure placed on Kizzy by professionals to abort her baby, and states:

> Having personal experience of dealing with the relevant services, we can tell you that it does appear to be geared-up to refer these young people for the obvious termination option.[17]

---

[15] Paignton Community and Sports College, 'Information to Parents of New Pupils 2006'.
[16] Personal correspondence, 26 June 2007.
[17] *ibid.*

Kizzy's pregnancy was not an isolated occurrence at the College which prides itself on its daily confidential advice service. Her mother writes:

I can categorically state that since December there have been four of her friends that have undergone terminations and a further two that have had or are due to have babies this year, not counting Kizzy.[18]

In spite of all the bold claims made about the 'success' of the TIC-TAC scheme, Kerry Neal notes that it has never been subjected to a proper independent evaluation.

Advocates of confidential services claim that they must be beneficial because without the guarantee of confidentiality young people would not seek advice. However, the question needs also to be asked whether young people might be less likely to engage in sexual activity in the first place in the absence of confidentality policies. It is worthy of note that in the United States teenage conception and abortion rates have declined more rapidly in areas where mandatory parental notification laws have been in place, prohibiting the supply of contraception and EHBC to underage young people without the involvement of parents.[19]

In the UK, however, there is a strong resistance even to questioning the merits of confidentiality policies. The Department of Health's revised guidance on confidentiality contains no acknowledgement of the law lords' ruling that contraceptive provision to underage girls without parental knowledge or consent should be 'most unusual' and occur 'only in exceptional circumstances', and its press release included a quote from Dr Vivienne Nathanson, the Head of Science and Ethics at the BMA, stating that:

it is essential that competent young people's autonomy continues to be recognised and respected in this way, to ensure a good doctor-patient relationship, based on trust, within which young people feel they are able to seek advice.[20]

However, in its attempt to enhance the trust between medical professionals and underage patients, the guidance is effectively breaking down the trust between parents and their children, which is a far more important relationship to safeguard. Parents are the primary protectors

---

[18] *ibid.*

[19] Levine P B, 'Parental involvement laws and fertility behavior', *Journal of Health Economics*, 2003: 22, 861-78.

[20] Department of Health press release, 'Publication of revised guidance for health professionals on the provision of contraceptive services to under 16s', 30 July 2004.

of their children, yet they are being sidelined in the name of 'the right of the child to confidentiality'. Vulnerable children and young people are increasingly being regarded and treated as autonomous individuals rather than members of a family, and parental responsibilities are being usurped by those whose interest in them is professional rather than personal.

Sue Axon's legal challenge

A High Court judgment in January 2006 confirmed that children are entitled to keep their parents in the dark concerning their pursuit of contraception, EHBC, abortion, and treatment for STIs. Manchester mother Sue Axon had argued that government guidance emphasising 'the duty of confidentiality' did not rest on a solid legal foundation and that medical professionals were under no obligation to provide such treatment to children without the knowledge of their parents unless to do so would prejudice the child's physical or mental health. However, Mr Justice Silber ruled that the Department of Health guidance was not illegal and was fully consonant with the 1985 law lords' ruling in the case brought by Victoria Gillick.

The 25,000-word judgment contains not a single reference to the age of consent to sexual intercourse, and does not appear to entertain the possibility that the existence and promotion of confidentiality policies might serve as an incentive to young people to become sexually active.

No account is taken of the fact that there was no significant change in the under-16 conception rate following Victoria Gillick's victory in the Court of Appeal, suggesting that the absence of confidentiality policies served not only as a disincentive to some young people to seek contraceptive advice, but also resulted in a reduction in underage sexual activity. Neither does the judgment give any weight to the evidence placed before the Court that demonstrates how teenage conception rates have declined more rapidly in areas within the United States where mandatory parental notification laws have been in place.

The Judge also appears to have been influenced by the support of many professional bodies for confidentiality policies for under-16s. For example, he noted that:

> [T]here is a generally held view within the BMA and other professional bodies that a duty of confidentiality is owed by a medical professional to a young person.[21]

and,

> There is additionally cogent evidence that doctors also clearly appreciate the importance of confidentiality to young people, who are considering seeking guidance on sexual matters.[22]

Having noted that approximately a third of abortions performed on girls under the age of 16 are carried out without the knowledge of either parent, the High Court ruling insists that:

> it remains the initial and significant duty of the medical professional to try to persuade the young person to inform his or her parents or to allow the medical professional to inform his or her parents.[23]

The judgment also rejects the contention of the *fpa* to the effect that it can no longer be assumed that parents are the best people to advise their children. At the very outset, the Judge ruled that it should be regarded as the norm to require the consent of a parent or guardian before providing surgical or medical treatment to a child aged under 16.[24]

Describing it as a 'very unfortunate situation' for a young person to seek advice without parental knowledge, the Judge was at pains to stress that:

> there is nothing in this judgment, which is intended to encourage young people to seek or to obtain advice or treatment on any sexual matters without first informing their parents and discussing matters with them... After all, the best judges of a young person's welfare are almost invariably his or her parents.[25]

The government's schizophrenic attitude

In recent years the government has adopted what can only be described as a schizophrenic attitude towards parents. While on the one hand it trumpets the importance of parents and holds them responsible for their

---

[21] R (Axon) v Secretary of State for Health [2006] EWCA372006 (Admin), para 42.
[22] ibid, para 68.
[23] ibid, para 101.
[24] ibid, para 1.
[25] ibid, para 2.

children's behaviour at school and in the community, on the other hand it undermines them by supporting measures such as the confidential provision of contraception, EHBC and abortions without their knowledge or consent.

After figures were published showing a rise in the number of conceptions to 13-15 year-old girls in 2005, the Minister for Children was swift to speak about the vital role of parents:

> We really need parents to now see themselves as making an absolutely unique and vital contribution to this issue... It is a contribution that I don't think anyone else can actually make.[26]

> We cannot make the deep, sustained progress we want to make, particularly at that vulnerable age group, without fully engaging with parents and getting them on board.[27]

Despite its rhetoric about the crucial role of parents, the government continues to pursue policies that undermine and marginalise them. Yet the more the state undermines the authority of parents, the less responsibility parents will be inclined to take for their children. Authority and responsibility go hand in hand. The government cannot have it both ways: it cannot disempower parents and at the same time blame them for society's ills. If the government wants parents to take proper responsibility for their children, it must first of all respect their authority.

---

[26] *The Guardian,* 26 May 2005.
[27] ePolitix.com, 27 May 2005
http://www.epolitix.com/EN/ForumBriefs/200505/a7c0a0a1-b4a4-48e0-a414-505e4c0f80c2.htm

9. The way forward

It is difficult to overestimate the confidence that has been placed in the free and confidential provision of EHBC to girls under the age of consent. Government ministers, Primary Care Trusts, doctors, nurses, schools – even Ofsted – never cease to sing its praises. If it has not delivered so far, then, it is argued, it needs to be made yet more readily accessible to children and young people by means of innovative and imaginiative initiatives. The possibility that it is destined to fail is never seriously contemplated. Schools are under pressure to make it available in on-site clinics, and pharmacists are strongly encouraged to raise public awareness of it and to promote its use. It has even reached the point where three-fifths of PCTs are prepared, in at least some circumstances, to refuse a pharmacy licence to applicants who have a principled policy of not supplying the emergency pill to girls under the age of 16.

PCTs

One might have thought that behind this widespread enthusiasm and growing pressure there would be a robust body of evidence demonstrating the effectiveness of EHBC to accomplish its twin purpose of reducing rates of unwanted pregnancy and helping the government achieve its targets in relation to teenage pregnancy rates. Yet research evidence did not feature in a single response to our survey of PCTs. Their policies appear to rest on the basis of assumption and wishful thinking rather than on hard facts.

Rather than persisting with an approach that is failing in the hope that it may 'come good' in the process of time, it is necessary for PCTs to undertake an honest appraisal of their policies in line with the evidence. Serious consideration needs to be given to the possibility that reliance on confidential access to contraception and EHBC may not be an effective way of reducing underage pregnancies, and may even be counterproductive in terms of the messages it sends out to children about casual sex, their exposure to the risk of STIs, and its impact on their relationships with their parents.

Those PCTs which do not currently have PGDs permitting the supply of EHBC to girls under the age of 16 should be in no hurry to introduce them, and those PCTs that do have such PGDs in place should review them in line with the evidence, and show more respect for the principled position of those applicants who have a policy of not supplying EHBC to underage girls. In the absence of any evidence that EHBC leads to a reduction in under-16 conceptions, it is untenable for PCTs to insist on supply to underage girls as a condition of granting a pharmacy licence.

Pharmacies

Pharmacies and supermarket chains that are currently supplying EHBC to girls under the age of 16 under a PGD also need to be made aware of the facts and encouraged to review their policies. They may be adding to the problem by giving the impression that they condone underage sexual activity and colluding with young people in keeping their parents in the dark rather than contributing to the solution.

Schools

As we have seen, the confidential provision of EHBC on school premises is incompatible with the government's own guidelines on the provision of drugs in schools, contravenes the guidelines given by the law lords in the 'Gillick' ruling; and undermines the responsibilities that parents bear towards their children. Headteachers and governing bodies need to be made aware of the issues at stake and encouraged to oppose the introduction of confidential health clinics in their schools. Where such provision has already been approved, it should be reviewed in line with the evidence.

Towards a better way

The failure of the government's teenage pregnancy strategy to meet its objectives has so far not prompted any serious examination of the methods being employed and their underlying assumptions. There are inevitably commercial interests that are resistant to considering an alternative approach, but that is not the only obstacle standing in the way of a radical re-evaluation of the teenage pregnancy strategy. Many of the bodies actively involved with promoting the confidential provision of contraception and EHBC to young people under the age of 16 are ideologically committed to supporting 'the right of the child' to engage in consensual sexual activity.[1]

There are, however, others who can see that the current approach is not working, but they persist with it because they simply do not know what else to do. If the answer to high teenage conception rates does not lie in more sex education and the promotion of contraception and EHBC, where does it lie? Advocates of contraception and EHBC provision to under-16s claim that the removal of such services would inevitably lead to increased conception rates, and many are persuaded by the argument that surely it is better to do something rather than nothing, even if the current approach is little more than an exercise in damage limitation.

The under-16 conception figures during the months following the Court of Appeal ruling in favour of Victoria Gillick at the end of 1984 place a question mark over such pessimistic predictions, and provide us with a clue to a more fruitful way forward.[2] The teenage pregnancy strategy is based on the premise that teenagers will continue to engage in sexual activity irrespective of anything parents and teachers say to them. The truth is, however, that the majority of young people under the age of 16 are not sexually active, and the evidence from the mid-1980s suggests that the sexual behaviour of a significant proportion of young people is influenced by the messages conveyed to them by public policy. The fact that under-16 attendances at family planning clinics went down by a third in 1985 while under-16 conception rates remained stable suggests that many underage girls who had previously been sexually active, or might have become sexually active if contraception had been available to them in confidence, chose to refrain from sexual activity.

Among sex education professionals in the UK there has been a surprising resistance to adopting an approach that supports and affirms the majority of under-16s in their exercise of self-control, and demonstrates to the minority the physical, emotional and psychological benefits

<hr/>

[1] See Riches V, *Sex Education or Indoctrination?* London: Family Education Trust, 2004.
[2] See chapter 5.

of saving sexual activity for marriage. While lip-service is paid to stressing the importance of 'the emotional side of relationships' in practice the emphasis is often on promoting 'safer sex' as a way of reducing the risk of unwanted pregnancies and the transmission of STIs. The idea of encouraging young people to save sex for marriage is dismissed as 'abstinence education', which its critics falsely claim amounts to nothing more than telling them to 'just say no'. However, until we overcome our current phobia about abstinence and our obsession with sexual expression, we are unlikely to make any real and sustained progress.

Index